Praise for *The Cleveland Clinic Guide to Menopause*

"Midlife women who are feeling betrayed by the unpredictability of their bodies and overwhelmed by the conflicting claims of the media will find clarity and empowerment in the pages of this book. Dr. Thacker demystifies menopause by using simple language to explain how the decline of estrogen levels can manifest itself as a broad array of symptoms, and she offers practical strategies for coping with those symptoms. The author acknowledges that each woman approaches menopause with a unique set of challenges—genetic risk factors, surgical history, medical issues, family stressors—and she invites the reader to explore different options for meeting those challenges . . . . This is an empowering message for women of all ages."

—ELIZABETH H. B. MANDELL, MD,
ASSOCIATE PROFESSOR, DEPARTMENT OF OBSTETRICS
AND GYNECOLOGY, UNIVERSITY OF VIRGINIA NAMS
CONSUMER EDUCATION COMMITTEE

"Dr. Thacker is the quintessential physician-advocate for women and our health. Her advice is sound, thorough, and easy to follow. Dr. Thacker empowers you to make good choices at so many levels."

—SYLVIA MORRISON,
MARKETING EXECUTIVE

"The Cleveland Clinic Guide to Menopause is rich with practical, scientifically grounded advice for healthy living. It's filled with sound strategies for dealing with the challenges of aging gracefully. This is a must-read that will help to empower women at midlife."

—WENDY KLEIN, MD, FACP,
ASSOCIATE PROFESSOR OF MEDICINE, OBSTETRICS & GYNECOLOGY,
VIRGINIA COMMONWEALTH UNIVERSITY SCHOOL OF MEDICINE,
AND DEPUTY EDITOR, *JOURNAL OF WOMEN'S HEALTH*

Also in the Cleveland Clinic Guide Series

The Cleveland Clinic Guide to

MENOPAUSE

Holly L. Thacker, MD

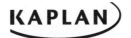

PUBLISHING

New York

Published by Kaplan Publishing, a division of Kaplan, Inc.
1 Liberty Plaza, 24th Floor
New York, NY 10006

Printed in the United States of America

10 9 8 7 6 5 4

Library of Congress Cataloging-in-Publication Data

Thacker, Holly.
  The Cleveland Clinic guide to menopause / Holly L. Thacker.
    p. cm. — (Cleveland Clinic guide series)
  Includes index.
  ISBN 978-1-4277-9970-8 (alk. paper)
  1. Menopause—Popular works. 2. Middle-aged women—Health and hygiene—Popular works. I. Cleveland Clinic Foundation. II. Title. III. Title: Menopause.
  RG186.T4786   2009
  618.1'75—dc22
                                                    2008047850

Kaplan Publishing books are available at special quantity discounts to use for sales promotions, employee premiums, or educational purposes. Please email our Special Sales Department to order or for more information at *kaplanpublishing@kaplan.com,* or write to Kaplan Publishing, 1 Liberty Plaza, 24th Floor, New York, NY 10006.

*It is my pleasure to dedicate this book to you, reader,
and to the thousands of women I've had the privilege of
treating during my years of practice of interdisciplinary
women's health.*

Contents

Introduction

You're a woman facing midlife. You care about your health, so you read the headlines and tune into the news programs. And if you miss the story of the day, you can count on a friend to fill you in. Daily "cutting-edge" reports spout the latest findings on women's health—breakthrough medications, warnings about hormone therapy, weight-loss fads, breast cancer rates. They seem to be talking directly to you.

Midlife can be a time to take stock of your health, feel invigorated, and plan for your "second adulthood." For many women, it is a marvelous time. But other women spend midlife barely staying afloat, frantically dog-paddling in a sea of turbulent symptoms that affect their work, health, sleep, mood, sex life, and happiness. And if that wasn't enough, they also have to deal with a barrage of mixed messages.

You may hear the new research that indicates low-fat diets won't prevent heart disease after all. Or you hear avoiding all carbs won't help you lose weight, all hormone therapy is dangerous, and those vitamins you're taking are even worse. One day your prescription is a medical miracle; the next, it's a killer. Talk about frustrating.

If all this were true or even partly accurate, being a woman today would be very risky business.

This should be the *best* time in history to be a midlife woman, thanks to the availability of so many safe and effective options for staying in good health. Instead I see droves of women suffering because alarmist reports have scared them away from proven, safe, effective treatments, and they're receiving erroneous information—and little support—from their doctors.

I see women weeping from fatigue after they've gone off hormone therapy because sheet-soaking nighttime hot flashes have robbed them of sleep and left them exhausted. I see depressed wives brought in by their husbands because their sex drive has vanished and they're enduring random panic attacks that make them feel they've lost control over their lives. I've seen women who have stopped effective osteoporosis therapies because they are petrified their jaws are going to drop off. In my twenty years of practicing medicine with a focus on hormone therapy and women's health at midlife, I haven't seen things as bad as they have been for menopausal women the past few years.

My daily contact with women, doctors, and students in training has shown me that too many people, both in and out of the medical field, have been receiving mixed messages about women's health issues. In spite of this, the specialty field of women's interdisciplinary and collaborative health care has come alive. I established our interdisciplinary Center for Specialized Women's Health at Cleveland Clinic in 2002, right about the time that the headlines were exploding with reports of the exaggerated dangers of hormone therapy.

When we opened the Center, I launched a "4HER" telephone hotline [(216) 444-4HER / (216) 444-4437], which women could call with their health concerns or questions.

And even though there are lots of books on the market focused on women and health (holistic health, menopausal health, bone health ... the list goes on), readers are still deprived of crucial information that could mediate their needless suffering and correct the distorted media claims and imprecise research surrounding women's midlife health issues.

This book provides that missing information.

In these pages, we will focus on vitality, health maintenance, hormones, hormone therapy, sleeping problems, cancer prevention, bone health, depression, panic attacks, heart health, sexual health, and the truth about vitamins and supplements, as well as some cutting-edge treatments for women's midlife health concerns.

If you've picked up this book, chances are that you'll recognize the struggles that some of my patients share as they cope with midlife. I hope that I can help dispel distorted media claims and inaccurate interpretations of research that mislead and confuse women and their physicians. Most of all, I hope reading this book will give you peace of mind and offer sound, practical information to help you regain control of your health during midlife. After all, it's your body, your hormones, and your choices.

By reading this book, you're taking the initiative for better health and renewed vitality. Congratulations! You're on your way.

Getting Answers

Each stage of life brings new changes and gives rise to new questions. We need answers that will help make our transitions smoother and guide us in maintaining a good quality of life. Unfortunately, we are often misled. The headlines don't spell out the whole story, and even in-depth reports leave out critical research conclusions—or jump to conclusions just to create media hype. The existence of so many variables can affect whether the results of a research study even apply to you. One study is just one piece of the puzzle. You need many pieces before you can see the big picture, much less complete it.

There is no doubt that the media is helpful. News programs and magazines make us realize how much research is out there, how many scientists, doctors, and patients are committed to finding answers so that women can live the healthiest, happiest lives possible. Many findings are inspiring, and more research is always on the way.

But the truth is, most women are confused. And who can blame them?

What's the *real* story? Whom can you trust to give you answers when those answers are constantly changing?

Within these pages, you'll find information on the following:

- Controlling menopause symptoms
- The truth about vitamins and supplements
- Diet and exercise to boost energy
- Bone health basics
- Myths and facts about hormone therapy
- Helping your heart in midlife
- Preventing cancer and other diseases
- Recharging your sex life
- Improving your vitality, longevity, and quality of life

Specialists like myself and others at the Cleveland Clinic's Center for Specialized Women's Health have dedicated our careers to studying, researching, and treating women's health issues. With so tight a focus, such doctors are better able to see that big picture— we have more of the puzzle pieces. The Cleveland Clinic Guides are designed to help you fit all the pieces of the puzzle together.

We're All Women, but We're All Different

You don't need a doctor to tell you we're all different. Just look at your mother, sisters, friends, and colleagues. So it should come as no surprise that there's no one-size-fits-all prescription that will calm raging hormones or restore balance during a time of life when change is the only constant.

It's a fundamental truth in women's health that there isn't a yes-or-no answer for every question, including these:

- Is hormone therapy a solution for every woman?
- Can you tell whether or not you'll experience a difficult menopause?
- Should you keep taking birth control in menopause?

- Are antidepressants a good idea?
- How can you stop hot flashes and get a good night's sleep?
- Are there hysterectomy alternatives?
- Can I get my sex drive back the way it was?
- Is surgery the best answer for a leaky bladder?

The media likes to categorize everything as good or bad, but with women's health, this just isn't possible. The only rules that apply to everyone are "Don't smoke," and "Wear your seat belt." That's about it. Even with diet, exercise, and vitamins, health recommendations will vary from person to person. We all need something different to look and feel our best.

Using the information gathered during physical exams and routine tests, ranging from blood-pressure readings to mammograms, is like playing a card game. Everyone gets a different hand because everyone's issues combine differently. The key is to develop a strategy based on the cards you're dealt. That's why it's critical to find a physician experienced in treating women's health issues.

It's also important to know the information you should have about your own health, the questions to ask your doctor, and the treatments available, both medical and holistic, that will enable you to maintain a vital lifestyle.

You need to build your knowledge. Invest in yourself by getting the straight facts about *you,* not your friend, neighbor, mother, or colleague.

A Strange Disconnect

When women come to see me the first time, they're usually eager to request the most complex, recently touted medical tests, but they don't seem to know the basics of everyday preventive health care. There's a disconnect between what women really *need* and what they ask for.

For example, many women have lately been asking for CA-125, a blood test that monitors ovarian cancer. This is a helpful tool for evaluating how a woman is responding to cancer treatment, but it is not a good screening test because it yields a high rate of "false positive" results and can miss many early cases of ovarian cancer. Sadly, I've seen many otherwise healthy women who had their healthy ovaries removed because the CA-125 results were elevated—not because of cancer but because of common, benign conditions like fibroids or endometriosis.

It baffles me when the same patient who asks for non-diagnostic ovarian cancer testing doesn't even know the symptoms of the disease, which she could be looking for herself. (Though subtle, there are signs you can watch for: pelvic pain, discomfort, and pressure; changes in bowel movements, such as frequency and consistency; frequent urination or a sudden urgent need to urinate; pain during sexual intercourse; abdominal pain, swelling, or a full or bloated feeling; persistent fatigue; weight gain around the abdomen; and sudden weight gain or weight loss.)

Most women don't know how to listen to their bodies. We haven't been trained in this relatively simple yet very important art. In addition, we haven't been given reliable information. For example, did you know that using the pill for five years can dramatically reduce your chances of getting ovarian cancer? Or that pregnancy also reduces risk? Do you know that it has been estimated that several cancer risks could be reduced 70 percent by optimizing vitamin D levels?

This is not to say that all women should take the pill or get pregnant, or dose themselves with vitamin D. Remember, there are no absolutes in women's health. Many educated women, even some who are doctors, are not aware of cancers and other diseases over which they have influence.

The point is that, while many patients ask for tests they've heard about on the Internet (like CA-125) that are usually not helpful, they neglect crucial, basic guidelines for good health.

This book will give you all the information you need to do everything you can to ensure your own good health and vitality. Then you'll be in the best position to make use of any screening tests and therapeutic treatments your doctor and you believe will help you live a long, enjoyable life.

It's All About Choices

They say that knowledge is power, but I'd make the case that the *right* knowledge is power. When we understand all our options, we can make better choices. We can gain control over our health, feel good about ourselves as our bodies change and mature, and enjoy our relationships more fully.

My goal is to share with you what we really know about the menopausal process, to dispel myths about treatment options like hormone therapy, and to discuss the many ways that you can maintain good health during midlife and improve areas of concern.

Midlife is the beginning of a time when most women can focus on their passions. You've spent years raising children; caring for a spouse; maintaining a career; and being a best friend, sister, and active community member. Now it's time to take care of number one—*you*.

Holly L. Thacker, MD, FACP, CCD
Director, Center for Specialized Women's Health
Women's Health Institute
Cleveland Clinic
www.clevelandclinic.org/womenshealth/
Associate Professor of Surgery, Cleveland Clinic Lerner College
    of Medicine at Case Western Reserve University
Executive Director, Speaking of Women's Health
www.speakingofwomenshealth.com

Chapter 1

Choosing and Seeing a Doctor at Midlife

W omen are naturals when it comes to sharing. When we listen, we really hear. When we talk, we express our deepest worries and greatest joys and form real connections with our sisters, best friends, mothers, coworkers, and neighbors.

Our male counterparts might call these verbal exchanges nothing but chatter. But women know better.

And because we are so practiced in reaching out and discussing personal issues, of course we're able to find the support we need when we're worried about our health, right?

Not exactly. Does this sound familiar?

Ellen
I haven't slept an entire night in ages because of these hot flashes. If this keeps up, I don't know how I'll manage to keep my job. And with my daughter's wedding coming up in three months, not to mention Mom's knee replacement, I'm not sure there will be enough of me to go around.

I was wondering whether hormone therapy would help. I decided to ask my next-door neighbor. After all, she's already been through this.

Well, Judy said she never took hormones during menopause, since their safety seemed questionable. And she doesn't seem any the worse for wear. In fact, she seems happy and healthy. And the way she and her husband behave, you'd think they were honeymooning! Now in my bedroom, on the other hand . . .

Yes, emotional support is just what women need. In fact, there is research to show that women with strong friendships and support systems recover from illness better than women who are more isolated. You simply can't put a price tag on the value of human connection and empathy. Hearing an affirming "Me too!" from a best friend might be just the thing that pulls you out of a funk.

But that's not *all* you need.

The right answer for your neighbor may not be the right answer for you. Judy never took hormones, yet she enjoys a great sex life. Nonetheless, hormones may alleviate *your* menopausal symptoms, as they did for Ellen, allowing her to participate in her daughter's wedding preparations, support her mother after her surgery, sleep better and therefore perform better at work, and just as important, ignite some of the missing mojo in the bedroom.

Go ahead and talk with friends and family. Get all the emotional support you need. But when you're seeking medical advice, don't leave your doctor out of the picture. After all, Mother (even your mother) doesn't always know best.

But where can you find a doctor you can trust, one who is knowledgeable about the ins and outs of women's health at midlife? I wrote this book in large part because I was so dismayed that smart women were seeing otherwise good doctors who gave them inaccurate information about women's health options.

Finding a Doctor

I can't stress strongly enough the fact that women are different. We have different needs from those of men, children, and even one another. And during the time from peri- to postmenopause, starting around age 40, we may need a physician specialist who can address the concerns unique to us.

Is My OB-GYN Enough?

Many women obtain all their health care, or all their woman-specific health care, from their OB-GYN. This seems to make sense—after all, OB-GYNs specialize in women's health, don't they? Depending on the nature of their medical practices, primary care doctors and OB-GYN physicians may or may not focus specifically on the health concerns of midlife women. Some women's health specialists (such as North American Menopause Society [NAMS] credentialed menopause specialists, for example) may have the knowledge, experience, or resources that you need.

So whom should you trust with your health? Well, that depends.

Should I See a Specialist?

If you have significant peri- or postmenopausal symptoms, such as panic attacks, hot flashes, or sexual problems that disrupt your life, or serious health disorders including osteoporosis, you may want to consider making an appointment with a physician who concentrates on women's health during midlife (i.e., menopause). His or her practice should encompass a knowledge of the following:

- Menopause and hormone therapy (HT)
- Bone health

- Sexual health
- Pelvic exams and Pap smears
- Urinary incontinence
- Mammograms and breast health
- Nutrition and exercise
- Mood disorders

Because menopause is a normal life stage, some women imagine that they must be weak if they need extra help. But this couldn't be further from the truth! After all, pregnancy and delivery are natural life stages, and most women seek professional support, education, and sometimes even medical intervention during those stages.

It's especially important to see a women's specialist if

- you have a personal or family history of breast or ovarian cancer.
- you have experienced blood clots.
- you've had previous adverse reactions to medicines.
- you have a personal or family history of hormonal upheaval.
- you've been told you have to have a hysterectomy and have had no other options discussed.

Strong women take control of their health, and that means seeking specialists who can provide the support and treatment options needed. Just because providers say they specialize in women's health and hormone therapy doesn't mean they actually have credentials. Many shady providers have seized on the opportunity to profit from women's misery and confusion. Be wary of any providers who sell you supplements, concoctions, and compounded hormones that they directly profit from, all the while falsely reassuring you that their personalized therapies are totally "natural" and "risk-free."

What Can I Expect From a Good Doctor?

Many women hit their emotional and physical peaks at midlife and breeze through menopause. Some make such a seamless transition that they don't even realize they're going through menopause.

But most of the women I see are not this lucky. Their lives have been thrown way off balance as they enter midlife. Take Cheryl, for instance.

Cheryl

Cheryl's husband of twenty-three years brought her in for an appointment. He didn't know what else he could do to support her.

She was falling apart, but you'd never know it from just a casual glance. Her appearance was flawless. She was dressed in an elegant pantsuit, and she looked healthy. But her eyes told a different story.

Once in my office, she described the symptoms she was experiencing. They turned out to be worse than what most women experience. Escalating mood swings abruptly nose-dived into emotional crashes, making her feel completely out of control. Her hot flashes were so sudden and substantial that she would find herself completely soaked in sweat. Her sex life was suffering tremendously, she said, because her vagina had virtually shriveled up. This was especially upsetting to her because she and her husband shared a deep love and had previously enjoyed an active sex life. As she was telling me all this, she broke down and sobbed.

It turned out that Cheryl's previous doctor had prescribed hormone therapy to restore hormonal balance and control her symptoms. The treatment worked well, but the doctor later pulled her off the drug in response to controversial reports in the medical and lay press. For Cheryl, stopping the treatments was the worst choice possible.

Red Flag

Be wary if your health care provider imparts absolutes. Women's health issues are never black and white. Answers to critical questions, such as the following, depend on the individual:

- "When should I get a mammogram?"
- "What kind of breast imaging is best for me?"
- "Is HT the only answer to treating menopausal symptoms?"
- "Is my depression due to menopause?"

These questions do not always have a simple yes-or-no answer. Every woman needs individualized options, education, and support. If your doctor gives you simplistic answers, move on. You deserve better.

Granted, Cheryl's case is somewhat extreme. The severity of her complaints is uncommon, but to one degree or another, most women experience similar symptoms.

No matter what physician you choose, she or he should be thorough and caring in discussing and exploring your symptoms, whether these are severe or more moderate.

During an initial appointment with a woman at midlife, I ask a lot of questions. This allows the patient to express her concerns and difficulties. I tend to ask questions in layers, first touching on health history and then progressing to menopause symptoms, if any. If these symptoms seem especially disruptive, I dig deeper.

From these questions and a full physical examination, I can generally spot indications that a woman is suffering unnecessarily.

Here are the questions I typically ask:

- At what age did you have your first menstrual period?
- When did you give birth to your first child?

- If you had a baby, did you breast-feed?
- Have you had a breast biopsy? Do you have a family history of breast or ovarian cancer?
- When did you have your last ThinPrep Pap test with HPV (human papillomavirus)test? Cholesterol ratios? Fasting blood sugar? Mammogram? Colon cancer screening? Bone density test?
- If you're menopausal, what is your history? When did your periods stop? Are you having menopause symptoms? Have you had any abnormal bleeding?
- What conventional or alternative treatments (such as vitamins, herbs, and supplements) are you taking?
- What are your sleep patterns? Do you have trouble falling or staying asleep? When you wake up, do you fall asleep again quickly?
- Do you have trouble breathing at night or snore badly? Do you notice shortness of breath during the day? Do you have heart palpitations?
- Do you experience hot flashes or flushing?
- Is your vaginal area dry?
- Have you noticed changes in your hair, skin, or nails?
- What about changes in bowel movements or bladder habits?
- How is your sex life?
- What is your mood and energy level on most days?
- Have you lost pleasure in activities you previously enjoyed?
- Do you feel anxious or depressed?
- Do you notice that your anxiety or depression changes with your menstrual cycle?
- Do you have a personal or family history of fibroid problems or hormonal upheaval?

- Did you ever experience postpartum depression or severe premenstrual syndrome (PMS) or bipolar disorder?

A patient's answers to these questions help me separate classic menopausal symptoms from medical conditions, psychiatric problems, or lifestyle issues such as being under stress from raising teenagers, caring for aging parents, or having pressures at work.

It can be challenging to tease out what symptoms are hormone related from those caused by mental health or environmental stressors. A thorough physical examination and questions such as these offer an excellent start.

Routine Tests and Screenings

When caring for a woman in midlife, a physician should perform a number of tests and screenings on a regular basis. If you have chosen a new physician, getting what are called "baseline" scores on these tests will allow her or him to establish what is normal for you. Knowing your scores allows the doctor to track any improvements or declines over the months or years between visits. (For more information on preventive health practices and other tips for midlife women, see appendix 1.)

Here are the tests you need.

Mammogram

Why? To screen for breast cancer. A diagnostic mammogram should be ordered if you or your physician identify some change or abnormality in the breast. It may involve spot views or magnification views of the breast and may include ultrasound. The breast radiologist is present during the test.

Many women get "called back" for a diagnostic mammogram. If this happens to you, don't panic. Most times, this is just for the breast imager to get a better picture of the breast. Digital mammography may be a better choice for women who are menstruating and/or who have denser breasts, as the image can be clearer.

How Often? Annually after age 40. The best time to have a mammogram is just *after* you've had your period or taken any progesterone. (This is because your breasts are most stimulated and tender when your progesterone levels are elevated, as they are during the second half of your menstrual cycle right before your period or when you have taken progesterone.)

Bone Density

Why? To measure the strength and density of bones, which provide early signs of osteoporosis.

How Often? Within two years of menopause; earlier for patients with a family history of osteoporosis, those who have previously broken or fractured bones, those who smoke, and those who have had low calcium and vitamin D intake.

Colonoscopy

Why? To screen for colon cancer.

How Often? Every five to ten years after age 50.

Blood Pressure

Why? High blood pressure increases the risk of stroke and heart disease.

How Often? Annually with your physician and at least monthly at home if you have high blood pressure. You can purchase a home blood pressure monitor at any drugstore. Digital monitors that strap around your biceps work the best.

Cholesterol

Why? High cholesterol levels are linked to obesity, heart attack, stroke, and hardening of the arteries.

If your levels of cholesterol are borderline elevated, you might want to ask for a cardio-CRP or ultrasensitive (US) CRP, which measures inflammation levels. (If you are on any oral hormones, the US CRP test will be falsely elevated and not helpful).

How Often? Annually if elevated but if levels are normal, every five years. However, be sure to check your cholesterol within two years of menopause because levels tend to fluctuate at this time.

Fasting Blood Sugar

Why? To detect blood sugar levels and identify symptoms of diabetes.

How Often? Every three years, starting at age 45; earlier for patients with a family history of diabetes, gestational diabetes, and/ or having had a baby over nine pounds at birth.

TSH (Thyroid-Stimulating Hormone) Test

Why? To detect thyroid dysfunction.

How Often? Every five years; sooner for patients with high cholesterol, menstrual disorders, or mood problems. Those with known thyroid problems should be monitored more often, as your doctor recommends.

Human Papillomavirus (HPV) Test, ThinPrep Pap Test, and the Pelvic Exam

Why? To detect HPV, a sexually transmitted infection (STI). Some strains of this virus can cause cervical cancer. Other strains can cause genital warts. (For more on HPV, see page 11.)

What You Should Know About HPV

HPV is a sexually transmitted disease caused by the human papillomavirus. There are 100 types of HPV, more than 30 of them spread through sexual contact. Women who get HPV often don't know they have it because its symptoms are silent. As many as 80 percent of all women have been exposed to HPV by age 50. Luckily, in most people, the infection clears without problems. Those who remain persistently infected with HPV, however, are at risk for cervical cancer.

Genital HPV can be spread by skin-to-skin contact; there doesn't have to be an exchange of bodily fluids as there does with AIDS transmission. Unfortunately, condoms do not prevent all HPV transmissions.

Women with high-risk strains of HPV may have abnormal Pap tests. Those with low-risk types may have minor abnormalities in a Pap test or may have genital warts.

Though HPV is usually harmless, some types can cause cervical cancer if not detected in time. Having regular Pap tests is the best way to ensure that any precancerous changes to cells will be caught and treated early.

If a woman has a normal Pap but is persistently positive for a high-risk HPV strain, I will recommend a colposcopy, a microscopic view of the cervix, to allow direct observation of the cervix for examination and biopsy of any suspicious areas. This procedure can take place in the doctor's office.

In 2006, Gardasil—the first cervical-cancer vaccine, which protects against four strains of HPV—came on the market. It is given to girls age 9 and older—up to age 26—in a series of three injections over six months. The vaccine reduces the risk of contracting certain high-risk strains of HPV known to cause cervical cancer or genital warts.

The immunization should be completed at least six months prior to any sexual activity, and females who have been immunized still need to have regular gynecologic exams and periodic Pap smears. HPV has been associated with other cancers such as anal cancer, lung cancer, penile cancer, and throat cancer. Both females and males are being routinely immunized in Australia.

If you have always had normal Pap smears all of your life and are HPV negative, you may discontinue the Pap smear (scrape of the cervix) at age 65 as the at-risk area of the cervix (the opening of the cervix) is no longer susceptible to HPV infection. However, if you have HIV or have not been regularly screened, you should continue with periodic Paps. All women, regardless of age or condition, need to continue with periodic exams.

How Often? Pap smears should begin within three years of commencing sexual activity or by age 21, whichever comes first. Pelvic exams with a Pap smear should be done yearly until age 30.

If you're over age 30, you should have both the ThinPrep Pap Test (a new form of the Pap test) and the HPV DNA test. If you've never been tested, ask about the test at your next doctor's visit.

If you're under age 30 and you've had an abnormal Pap test, be sure to get tested for HPV.

Regardless of your age, get tested every three years after your initial test. Also, if you carry the high-risk HPV, you'll need more frequent Pap smears, age again notwithstanding. Conversely, if you're over age 30 and you've had normal Pap smears, you can safely space your Pap smears to every three years. However, you should still get a yearly pelvic exam.

If you've had a hysterectomy for benign, noncancerous reasons, you no longer need a Pap smear of the cervix because the cervix is no longer present. However, you still need a periodic pelvic exam. And if you were exposed to DES (diethylstilbestrol) in utero, you must continue with yearly Pap smears regardless of cervical and HPV status.

I also recommend getting a clean bill of health, including a pelvic exam, ThinPrep Pap Test, and cervical cultures, if you have changed sexual partners.

Shared Medical Appointments

Once you've had your initial visit with your doctor and gotten all your tests and screenings, you might enjoy a new approach to follow-up care, the shared medical appointment (SMA). This arrangement groups together about ten women who return to the doctor's office at the same time for test results, follow-up care, and information on the latest developments in women's health. They meet in a comfortable lounge and speak with a behavioral-health counselor and, of course, their physician.

Test results and further follow-up suggestions are given to each woman individually, while the others learn about new treatment options with a focus on lifestyle and diet.

The women who have tried this style of appointment at our Center for Specialized Women's Health seem to enjoy it. They spend ninety minutes with the doctor instead of five or ten, and they're able to connect with other women dealing with the same health problems as their own.

If your health care facility offers this arrangement, it could be highly beneficial for you. (See appendix 2 for more information.)

On the Record: Maintaining Your Own File

My final suggestion on making the most of your doctor visit is to give you an assignment. A great way to stay in charge of your own health is to keep a detailed medical file at home. Just as you maintain financial records and even details on when your car was last serviced, you should keep your own medical file.

If you don't have your records on hand, you're like most patients—even nurses and doctors—who don't know their cholesterol level, how much vitamin D they are taking, or even whether one or both of their ovaries were removed during a hysterectomy.

This kind of information is vitally important, especially if you switch doctors or move to a new city. While technology and online medical records look promising, for now we all need to take responsibility for keeping hard copies of our medical records. I advise all my patients to keep track of the important markers of health. It's also important to keep records, as you never know when a computer virus will "eat" vital information.

Some of these practices are probably already habits for you. I'll bet you weigh yourself regularly and know when (or if) you'll be getting your menstrual period. But do you write down this information and track it on a calendar or in a log? Now is the time to start.

Why bother to keep a health file? Weight and height, for example, determine your body mass index (BMI), an important factor in determining your risk for certain conditions such as heart disease. Similarly, knowing the dates of your past menstrual cycles can help you and your doctor determine whether you have started menopause.

So designate a special file where you can keep personal records, along with information provided by your doctor. Pick out a pink folder. Make it hot pink, even—something that stands out. Listed below is the kind of information you should collect. Be sure to keep it somewhere handy; don't stick it behind other files or in the bottom of a drawer.

Bring your folder to every visit with your doctor. Take the time before the appointment to review your latest records and be sure to note any questions or concerns you want to bring up at the visit.

Keeping track of your records allows you and your doctor to plan the optimum course of prevention or treatment together.

What Should I Keep Track of in My File?

Compile these important statistics and make sure you keep hard copies that you update regularly.

Weight. Weigh yourself once a week and keep this information on a calendar or chart. Avoid hopping on the scale each day—weighing yourself shouldn't become an obsessive activity. Choose the same day and time of day every week (for example, Wednesday mornings).

We all know that the scale will tip after an indulgent weekend or during a certain time of the month or even throughout the day. Our weight can fluctuate several pounds throughout the week, so weigh yourself weekly in the morning. Don't let numbers determine your mood—or your dinner plans.

Why is weight important? Overweight women generally have higher cholesterol levels and higher blood pressure. These increase the risk for heart disease and diabetes. Increased weight contributes to other medical problems as well, such as arthritis, obstructive sleep apnea, gallbladder disease, and certain cancers.

Ultimately, weight gain also affects quality of life, including the way you look and feel each day.

Height. Most women "shrink" with age, in height if not in weight. How many inches we lose can be a sign of our skeletal health (bone density).Weak bones of lower density eventually translate into osteoporosis, a more full-fledged bone loss that results in painful fractures, which can curtail lifestyle and even lead to death.

So get in the habit of measuring yourself. Many of us don't know our true height. You should be measured yearly.

Body Mass Index. Women are more prone to weight gain than men because female hormones tend to promote fat formation. Our bodies simply store fat more easily. What's more, the muscle mass we lose after age 40 (in a process known as sarcopenia) is often replaced with body fat. The older we get, the harder we have to work to fight the fat because the metabolism slows.

BMI, or body mass index, is a reliable indicator of total body fat, which is related to your risk of disease and death. BMI is a measure of your weight relative to your height and waist circumference.

Calculating your BMI gives you a good idea of whether you need to control your weight better to fight disease risk or whether you fall within a healthier normal range.

To calculate your BMI, take your weight in pounds, divide by your height squared, and multiply by 703.

For example, let's find the BMI of a woman who is five feet five inches tall and weighs 155 pounds. Her weight, 155, needs to be divided by her height, squared. To square her height, it must first be calculated in inches: 12 inches (in a foot) × 5 (feet) + 5 (more inches) = 65 inches. This number then gets multiplied by itself: 65 inches × 65 inches = 4,225. So now we have 155 to be divided by 4,225. This equals 0.037. The last step is to multiply 0.037 by 703, which equals 26.0. So, in our example, this woman's BMI is 26.0 or "borderline." (See the table.) What's yours?

BMI	WEIGHT STATUS
Below 18.5	Underweight
18.5–24.9	Normal
25–27	Borderline
27.1–29.9	Overweight
30 and above	Obese

Our mythical woman with the BMI of 26.0 is not really overweight but not quite normal weight, either. This is the most important time to do more intensive exercise and engage in healthy eating habits to prevent further weight gain. It is much easier to prevent obesity than to treat it.

Bear in mind that a BMI score does have some limits. Athletes and individuals with a muscular build will have a higher BMI. Older people who have lost muscle mass will have a lower BMI. Talk to your doctor about your individual result.

Family History. You can't choose your genes, but you can take steps to mitigate your risk of cancers, diseases, and other medical conditions that run in your family. If your mother had breast cancer, your risk of getting it is greater than that of a woman with no family history. It helps if you know things like how old your mother was when she entered menopause. Did your grandmother have osteoarthritis or break a hip?

The more you know, the more you can control your future health.

Vitamins, Supplements, and Prescription Medications. Know what medications, vitamins, and supplements you're taking and what the dosages are. Bring the bottles to your doctor appointment.

Many women don't mention herbal remedies and nonprescription treatments when doctors ask about medication use. But these can have a significant impact on other medications, health conditions, and even anesthesia if you're having surgery. So remember to speak up about these.

Fasting Cholesterol Levels. Cholesterol ratios change before and right after menopause; the same goes for blood pressure. Knowing your cholesterol is important for identifying risk for heart disease, diabetes, and stroke. Your doctor can give you a referral to a laboratory where they will test your blood. You may also be able to get your cholesterol checked at health fairs or local drugstores.

Blood Pressure. The guideline for women is 115/75, and many of my patients exceed this.

I recommend checking your blood pressure in the morning, as it tends to be a bit higher then. It's also good to check your blood pressure under different circumstances, such as during relaxation, after physical exercise, or when you're feeling stress.

If you continue to log high blood pressure readings, don't wait until an annual checkup to do something about it.

What Does My Blood Pressure Reading Actually Mean?

A healthy heart beats in a predictable cycle, first contracting to send blood out to the body, then relaxing to refill with blood for the next push. The top number in your blood pressure reading indicates the "systolic" pressure, the force of blood when the heart contracts. The bottom number, the "diastolic" pressure, represents the force of the blood in the vessels when the heart is at rest.

Some people have elevations of both systolic and diastolic blood pressure; some have elevation of only one. In either case, it's very important to control high blood pressure (also known as "hypertension").

Without treatment, high blood pressure can lead to the following:

- Stroke
- Enlarged heart
- Kidney disease
- Heart failure
- Heart attack
- Hemorrhages in the blood vessels of the eye
- Peripheral vascular disease.

I tell most of my patients to keep their blood pressure around 115/75. If yours is consistently higher, please contact your physician for advice.

Dates of Tests and Screenings. Make sure to save the results of all the tests discussed above. You can get copies from your doctor. You'll want to know the answers to these questions:

- When was your last bone density test?

- When was your most recent mammogram?

- When did you last have a fasting blood sugar test, Pap smear, colonoscopy, HPV screening, or TSH check?

- Are your immunizations all up-to-date? Have you had a tetanus booster in the last ten years? Have you had the new tetanus booster Tdap (Adacel), which covers tetanus, diphtheria, acellular pertussis, and whooping cough (which is making a comeback)?

- If you're over age 50, do you get your flu vaccine faithfully every fall? (You should!) If you're over age 60 (or younger but have chronic medical problems), have you had the pneumonia vaccine PNEUMOVAX? If you're over age 60 and have had chickenpox but have not yet had shingles, have you had ZOSTAVAX, the shingles vaccine?

Other Records. Along with your medical records, you might also want to save or make note of any useful health references you have or can find online or at the library, such as

- current guidelines for screening cancers;

- domestic (intimate partner) violence help-line information;

- power of attorney for health care;

- additional patient-education sheets; and

- select websites and recommended book titles (see appendix 6)

Ready to Roll

Now you know what you need to do to find a doctor, what questions to ask, what tests you need, what to expect, and how to keep track of your own health information.

You have the knowledge and the tools. You're ready to be a full partner in your health care.

Chapter 2

Symptoms
of Menopause

W hen they approach midlife, some women suddenly find themselves lost in an avalanche of debilitating symptoms that daily threaten their quality of life. Depression, anxiety, sleep loss—you name it. Menopause barrels into their lives like a runaway truck, damaging appearance, mood, sex life, and sense of self-worth. That's Kathy's predicament, and maybe it's yours, too.

Kathy

Everything in my life was falling into place like a Kodak moment. My two beautiful daughters announced their engagements, and our family—always so close—felt complete. We celebrated with gatherings whenever possible. My career allowed me more freedom to pursue hobbies I had put on hold for years, especially gardening, which I love. My husband and I even planned a postwedding cruise, anticipating the need for a break after a hectic year. The vacation would be a second honeymoon for us.

Our album of pictures from that year shows photographs of me smiling—beaming, even. Picture-perfect. I don't know how I held it together. Many days I didn't.

"Kathy just isn't Kathy," my sisters confided to each other. They were right. My periods had stopped, and my body had abruptly changed. My panic attacks were unpredictable and uncontrollable. Frighteningly, at night, a racing heartbeat shook my whole body. My legs and arms would go numb as I imagined myself in a wheelchair, my life crashing down around me. I headed to more than one emergency room and consulted several doctors.

Of course, my husband, Bill, loved me, comforted me, and held me. He knew I wasn't getting better, and neither of us could pretend differently.

I couldn't sleep, which made everything worse. I was still smiling and trying to hold it together for my daughters on the outside, but I was falling apart on the inside. How could a mother and wife be so distressed and feel so desperate during what was supposed to be a happy time?

I finally visited a physician who specialized in women's health. After conducting a complete physical exam, gynecological exam, hormonal assessment, and series of tests, she determined that my symptoms were associated with hormone fluctuations, the onset of menopause, and panic disorder, all very treatable conditions.

"You're kidding!" I said to her. Unbelievable. These symptoms were not the classic hot flashes I'd had heard about.

On a scale of one to ten for menopause symptoms, Kathy's case pushes the limit. Her situation is somewhat unusual, although no woman's experience while her reproductive system winds down could be classified as "normal." This goes back to my point that every woman is different; one woman may breeze through menopause, not realizing that she is officially "in menopause" until she counts off twelve menstruation-free months. Ta-da—a seamless transition. Her life is barely affected by "the change." Another may suffer the way Kathy did—until she received proper treatment, that is.

Menopause Is Natural

During this time, it's important to remember that *menopause is a natural part of aging. It is not a disease.* However, just as with menstruation and childbirth, an educated assessment and some medical attention may be necessary.

Many of my patients nearing their early 50s regard the years leading up to menopause (called perimenopause) as a living hell. But they don't have to be.

If your symptoms make you feel like the shell of the person you were just months ago, you're probably wondering "Why me?" The answer to this question is multifaceted. First, we must understand what happens inside a woman's body during the onset of menopause. Because menopause varies with every woman, knowledge is the best tool for maintaining a positive attitude.

The Inside Story

A woman's life can be divided into three hormonal phases, comparable to the acts in a play:

- Reproduction
- Menopause
- Postmenopause

The pituitary gland in the brain is the "director," telling the body how much of certain hormones to make during each of the three phases. Furthermore, current medical thinking recognizes that what most people refer to as "menopause" is actually a process involving three stages: perimenopause, menopause, and postmenopause.

What Is Perimenopause?

During this period, ovarian function becomes erratic. A woman may detect physical signs, such as hot flashes and irregular periods. Perimenopause usually begins sometime in a woman's 40s and lasts a full year after the final menstrual period.

What Is Menopause?

This is the time when the ovaries stop releasing eggs and a woman no longer has periods. Menopause usually occurs between the ages of 45 and 55. A general indication of menopause is cessation of periods for twelve consecutive months. The average age for women to experience menopause in this country is 51.3 years.

• • • *Fast Fact* • • •

The term *menopause* comes from the Greek *meno,* meaning month, and *pausis,* a pause or stop.

• • •

What Is Postmenopause?

The postmenopausal time frame is divided into early postmenopause—the first five years since the last menstrual period—and late postmenopause—five years and beyond. The early postmenopausal phase is the most critical in terms of symptoms and bone loss and is generally the time frame that hormone therapy is initiated if indicated. You can not base medical decisions on age alone; a 55-year-old woman could be ten years past menopause in the late postmenopausal phase, she could still be menstruating and be premenopausal, or she could be starting to skip menses and be perimenopausal or in the "menopause transition."

What's Causing All of This Change?

Our levels of estrogen, testosterone, and progesterone, the main characters in our cast of hormones, fluctuate throughout our lives. This up-and-down process sometimes produces happy endings. At other times, hormone imbalance creates conflict. And the plot thickens.

Estrogen. Estrogen is the term for a class of female sex hormones secreted by the ovaries. The three major kinds of estrogens are estriol, estradiol, and estrone.

Estrogen influences the development and maintenance of typical female sex characteristics, such as increased body fat in hips and thighs and smoother skin (compared to men). Estrogen also influences the female reproductive system in many ways, including preparing the body for reproduction.

Progesterone. Progesterone is a steroid hormone that prepares the uterus for pregnancy, maintains pregnancy, and promotes development of the mammary glands. The main sources of progesterone are the corpus luteum (formed after ovulation in the ovary) and the placenta.

The term *progestogens* encompasses both progestins (synthetic versions of the hormone) and progesterone itself.

Testosterone. Testosterone affects sex-related features and development. In men, it is produced in large amounts by the testicles. In both men and women, testosterone is also produced in small amounts by the adrenal glands and, in women, by the ovaries.

Estrogen Plays the Lead. Let's focus for a minute on the key hormone that signals menopause onset—our leading lady, estrogen. Before a woman goes into menopause, more than 90 percent of her estrogen is made by the ovaries. (Organs that make smaller amounts include the adrenal glands, the liver, and kidneys.)

Estrogen regulates your monthly cycles of ovulation and menstruation. It also plays a role in your psychological well-being, which covers your mood, sleep, and sex drive; your urinary tract; your skin and vaginal tissues; and your bones and heart. In addition, estrogen is involved in your blood-vessel tone and the health of your gums, teeth, and eyes.

Historically, estrogen has been "typecast" as the girls-only hormone, regarded for its role in women's reproductive functions. It is applauded for helping to bring babies into the world and for creating women's attractive hourglass figures—sometimes it's blamed when those figures keep us from fitting into our favorite jeans.

Estrogen is all woman. And, like women, estrogen has a brainy side.

Estrogen affects the brain's blood flow. It can boost verbal memory (testosterone supports spatial memory) and improve the way the brain processes information. Estrogen can also affect mood. For example, decreased estrogen levels can affect serotonin levels, which in turn can spark anxiety and/or depression. This explains why a woman with no medical history of depression may go through a bout just as she enters menopause.

• • • *Fast Fact* • • •

It's ironic that the average 55-year-old man may have a higher estrogen level than the average 55-year-old woman. That is because men usually enjoy steady testosterone production as they age, and testosterone is regularly converted into small amounts of estradiol/estrogen. But a woman suffers from decreased estrogen production as she enters menopause. A woman who loses her ovaries or her eggs no longer has a constant source of estradiol production.

• • •

Short-term Symptoms

When your ovaries stop making estrogen, you go into menopause, and your periods end. For all intents and purposes, estrogen has left the stage.

But as we've just seen, estrogen isn't involved only in your reproductive system. Other body systems are affected by estrogen levels, too, so it's easy to understand why menopause gets its tentacles into so many areas of physical, mental, and emotional function.

Unfortunately, we usually don't realize how important estrogen is to maintaining physical and mental balance until we are running on empty. Then, strange symptoms often suggest that something different is going on in the body.

Here's a list of common menopausal symptoms:

- **Hot flashes.** Sudden sensations of heat that spread from the chest to head, often followed by sweating and cold shivering. A hot flush is not the flash but the redness that suffuses the neck and face. (See chapter 7 for more about hot flashes.)

- **Night sweats.** Hot flashes that occur during sleep and cause perspiration.

- **Difficulty sleeping.** Often related to hot flashes and night sweats.

- **Vaginal changes.** These include dryness and increased vulnerability to bladder infections.

- **Sex drive.** Mood changes can affect a woman's interest in sex, as can vaginal dryness, making sex more uncomfortable.

- **Mood changes.** These can include irritability, anxiety, and mood swings.

- **Skin changes.** These include dryness, itching, and loss of elasticity.

- **Headaches/migraines.** These may be worsened by hormone fluctuations, although migraines usually get better after menopause. (For more information on migraines, see appendix 3.)

- **Heart palpitations.** These can be manifestations of symptoms (such as hot flashes) in the autonomic system (the nerves and muscles that cause the blood vessels to constrict or dilate), but any heart symptom needs to be checked out by a doctor before being attributed to menopause.

- **Hair.** Increased facial hair or thinning hair on the head can be due to lack of estrogen and/or increased sensitivity to remaining testosterone.

- **Memory loss/poor concentration.** Forgetfulness or reduced ability to think clearly can be related to hormone fluxes, lack of sleep, increased stressors, undiagnosed medical problems, vitamin deficiencies, or depression.

Age-related Changes

For all women, aging and menopause go hand in hand—so, naturally, the estrogen loss of menopause is linked to a number of health problems that are considered common signs of aging. After menopause, women are more likely to suffer from the following:

- **Changes in bladder function.** These can be age related, or they can result from genetic predisposition, childbearing trauma, or weight gain. (Bladder function can become more overactive with the loss of estrogen.)

- **Poor brain function.** This includes an increased risk of Alzheimer's disease associated with advanced age.

- **Loss of skin elasticity.** This results in increased wrinkling.

- **Decreased muscle tone and bone loss.**

- **Some changes in vision.**

- **Weight fluctuation and slower metabolism.**

Some women feel defeated when they confront these issues. We can't stop the clock, after all. But you can control many of these problems with relative ease by eating well, exercising regularly, protecting the skin from sun damage, taking the right vitamins and supplements, and staying actively involved in life as you work with your physician to design a personalized regimen. (We'll talk more about age versus hormones in chapter 3.)

Long-term Problems

There are long-term risks that women inherit with age and menopause. Heart disease and osteoporosis are two of the most serious. The heart and bones can suffer tremendously from estrogen deficiency, making it especially important to take measures to reduce cholesterol, lower blood pressure, refrain from smoking, and maintain bone mass.

Fortunately, lifestyle choices can modify these risks. We will discuss these and other ways to reduce these risks throughout this book.

Are We There Yet?

Estrogen doesn't usually vanish from your body all at once, without warning.

Decline in estrogen starts during perimenopause, the phase before full-blown menopause. During perimenopause, hormones begin to fluctuate, periods may occur at unpredictable intervals, and bleeding may be quite heavy and periodically hormone levels can surge.

Perimenopause usually begins in a woman's 40s, sometimes lasting as long as eight to ten years. This does *not* mean that over this entire period you will notice signs of the onset of menopause. It simply means that your ovaries are winding down their ovulatory function. In fact, you may not recognize any of the short-term symptoms we just discussed until you reach the last few years of perimenopause, when estrogen production drops more dramatically and more quickly.

Perimenopause lasts until menopause, when the ovaries stop releasing eggs completely.

How Can I Tell That I've Reached Menopause?

When a woman stops having her menstrual period and hasn't had one at all for twelve months, she is medically defined as menopausal. (We'll talk more about breakthrough or abnormal bleeding in chapter 13.)

How old you are when you experience menopause is related to the number of eggs in your ovaries, which is determined by a genetic component. If the women in your family generally go into menopause in their early 40s, chances are that you'll experience an early menopause, too.

Your lifestyle and medical history also can affect the age you'll be when you go into menopause. For example, smokers and women with chronic illness are more likely to experience early onset.

In certain cases, women may enter menopause without knowing it or can even experience induced menopause.

Can I Be Tested for Menopause?

Everyone wants a "menopause test," something that will predict when menopause will actually happen, but testing for menopause is a bit trickier than checking body temperature or diagnosing strep throat.

Red Flag

If a woman is over 50 years old, has gone even six months without a period (an indication of the onset of menopause), and then bleeds or spots, she should see a doctor within that month.

This kind of postmenopausal bleeding is often caused by treatable and relatively benign conditions. But in some cases—perhaps up to 5 percent—postmenopausal bleeding can indicate uterine cancer or a precursor, such as hyperplasia (an abnormal increase in cells).

If you do experience such bleeds or spots, you should get a Pap smear, pelvic exam, special saline-infusion sonogram (SIS), and an endometrial sampling, in which the doctor takes a biopsy, or small sampling, of the endometrium (the lining of the uterus) to examine.

For more on abnormal bleeding and what to do about it, see chapter 13.

The best way to confirm menopause is by analyzing symptoms associated with estrogen deficiency and performing a thorough history and physical exam, including the following:

- **Determination of menstrual patterns.** These include your age, menstrual history, and the number of months that you have missed your period, as well as the appearance of such classic symptoms as hot flashes.

- **Assessment of vaginal tissues.** The major indicator of menopause is the condition of the vaginal tissues, which are the body tissues most sensitive to estrogen loss. Normally, the vagina is thick, plush, and pink. In estrogen-deficient women, the vagina is thin, pale, flat, and dry. It also becomes more alkaline. If the vaginal tissue is really thin, it may appear red and can tear and bleed easily.

- **Measuring bone density and bone tissue.** Bone is sensitive to the levels of estrogen and other hormone levels, and it may show density loss when estrogen production decreases over time.

Still, many patients insist on black-and-white test results, and many physicians perform lab tests that, while offering a momentary snapshot of the various hormone levels, are not really at all helpful in diagnosing or predicting menopause.

The following tests are *not* accurate ways of confirming menopause and do *not* paint a picture of total body estrogen:

- **pH test.** When estrogen levels fall, pH levels in vaginal tissue increase. Your doctor can measure the pH levels in your vagina with simple pH paper in the office, but this is not a foolproof confirmation of menopause because some vaginal infections also cause vaginal pH levels to rise.

- **Saliva tests.** Saliva contains a fraction of the hormones that are in the bloodstream. Most salivary tests are a waste of money and are not a valid way to measure levels of progesterone, or estradiol (a potent type of estrogen), and testosterone. And even when we do know a woman's level of estradiol, we cannot predict when she will run out of eggs and, therefore, lose most of her estrogen production. In addition, cigarette smoke, certain foods, hormone therapy or hormonal contraception, and environmental stressors can affect the results of saliva tests.

- **Urinary tests.** Urine tests promising to give indications of menopause onset can be purchased without a prescription for home use. These measure pituitary gonadotrophins, which are typically elevated in menopause. Again, these are not always reliable because these levels begin to elevate during the years before menopause, so it could be as long as ten years later when menopause begins. Be aware that, even with elevated urine-test results, if you haven't gone twelve months without a period, you could still be premenopausal or perimenopausal, and you're still at risk for pregnancy.

• **Follicle-stimulating hormone (FSH) test.** FSH tests measure blood levels of FSH. FSH rises each month to encourage follicles in the ovaries to release eggs, causing a menstrual period. A high FSH level may indicate that your body is working hard to release eggs and may not be unsuccessful. Depending on how high the levels are, this may indicate perimenopause or menopause. But FSH levels fluctuate considerably from one minute to the next, thus making them unreliable indicators of menopause. The test is usually ordered within the first three days of the period (when the levels should be at lower levels) and can be used during infertility evaluations to assess ovarian reserve.

Many doctors simply order these tests to satisfy women who demand a "menopause test," but they are neither predictive nor definitive.

Are Menopause- and Estrogen-related Tests Reliable?

Ultimately, body fluid (blood, saliva, and urine) tests are not the most accurate ways to measure estrogen levels in women. Metabolism is complex where estrogen is concerned. A woman may have a low level of estrogen in the blood but high levels in certain body tissues. What's in your bloodstream or saliva is not as important as what's in such body tissues as the brain, breasts, bones, or reproductive and urinary system.

Alone, these tests are not reliable indicators of menopause. However, paired with a clinical evaluation, bone density test, and thorough physical examination, they can serve as supporting evidence. Persistently elevated FSH levels usually imply impending menopause.

• • • *Fast Fact* • • •

Premature menopause occurs in less than 1 percent
of women under the age of 40. Reasons can range
from autoimmune conditions to fragile X syndrome
to chemotherapy treatment.

• • •

How Does Birth Control Affect Menopause?

In addition to its contraceptive uses, I sometimes prescribe the
pill to alleviate symptoms during perimenopause. But if you are
taking the pill, your periods won't tell you whether you're officially in menopause or not. (You still get periods when you're on
the pill, even if your body wouldn't naturally menstruate.) So how
do you know?

The only way to tell is to go off the pill. But keep in mind that
the timing of such an experiment is up to you. If you're dealing
with several heavy stressors in your life, it may not be the right time
to experiment with your hormone levels.

For example, take Valerie.

Valerie

*Valerie was a fifty-two-year-old patient of mine who asked me
if I thought she should stop taking the pill. She didn't need the
prescription for contraceptive purposes any more, since her husband had a vasectomy. However, she was finishing her master's
degree and juggling a demanding career while caring for her
ailing and elderly mother.*

*I asked her to consider whether this was really the best time
to introduce another potential stress into her life. She decided
to wait until she had earned her degree.*

What Is Hormonal Contraception?

Today, birth control comes in a variety of forms collectively known as "hormonal contraception," or HC. HC includes the pill, the patch, the vaginal ring, uterine devices, and subdermal (under-the-skin) implants.

Of course, Valerie might have gone off the pill and felt just fine. But it was equally possible that once she did so, her hormones would have proceeded to rage out of control or precipitously drop to very low levels.

Here's the bottom line: If you're on the pill and don't smoke, and have normal blood pressure and overall good health, it's usually safe to continue taking the pill until you reach age 55. And it's fine to pick a time when life is not taking you for a spin to test how you feel when you're not taking hormones.

During this time, I always talk with my patients about symptoms of menopause so they understand what to expect. Some of them go off the pill, never get another period, and suffer few if any symptoms. Others crash into menopause with severe side effects.

If a woman comes off the pill and ends up having difficult symptoms, I may put her back on it if she still needs contraception. Or I'll prescribe hormone therapy. I try again later to take her off the pill.

• • • *Fast Fact* • • •

Estrogen therapy is not a risky solution to menopausal symptoms for most women who have had hysterectomies.

• • •

Hysterectomy and Hormone Therapy

Women who have had hysterectomies do not have menstrual periods, but they can still produce hormones (estrogen) if one or both ovaries are intact. In a woman who has had a hysterectomy but still has her ovaries, when her estrogen levels fall, she may experience symptoms of menopause just like any other woman.

Sometimes women who have had hysterectomies begin menopause a few years earlier because of disturbance to this sensitive reproductive area.

Women who have both the uterus and ovaries removed during a hysterectomy are likely to experience the immediate onset of menopausal symptoms because their bodies no longer produce estrogen. (No ovaries, no estrogen.) This type of menopause is known as surgical or induced menopause, and it tends to be more severe.

Many women who have had hysterectomies ease into menopause without a problem. Without a uterus, most of these women no longer experience monthly bleeding or pain, and they generally enjoy fulfilling sex lives. But there are no absolutes.

One of every six to ten women whose ovaries were removed during a hysterectomy is thrown into a tailspin during menopause. Not only are her hormones out of balance, her body may be depleted of estrogen and testosterone. Hysterectomy surgery can cause a woman to lose most or all of her estrogen and as much as 25 to 50 percent of her testosterone sources.

For most women in this situation, hormone therapy is an effective treatment choice for the alleviation of severe menopausal symptoms. And there are many different ways to take HT, including pills, creams, gels, vaginal rings, and patches.

When physicians deny women in this condition the opportunity to take hormone therapy, it's like telling a woman who needs shoes that she should be able to get along with slippers or boots, or just go barefoot.

Is Menopause Easier With or Without Ovaries?

A hysterectomy is a major surgery to remove a woman's uterus, often performed to treat a health issue. The procedure may also include removal of other reproductive organs, including one or both ovaries, the fallopian tubes, and the cervix.

I advise my patients to keep their ovaries until at least age 65 unless there is good reason to remove them, such as cancer or the presence of one of the mutations of the breast cancer gene (BRCA genes), which indicates high risk for breast and ovarian cancer.

When women are shut out of proven options like hormone therapy, we lose our freedom of choice and the ability to decide which solution is best for us.

You need a doctor who is knowledgeable about the women's health field and who presents all the options. Not all family physicians and OB-GYNs keep up with the latest studies on hormone therapy. Doctors should know that estrogen therapy is not a risky solution for most women with hysterectomies. However, even medical professionals can be influenced by the media.

If you've had your ovaries removed during hysterectomy, be sure that your doctor is familiar with all the therapy options. There's no reason for you to suffer.

Chapter 3

What's to Blame, Age or Hormones?

For women, it isn't always clear whether a specific health symptom, such as weight gain or hair loss, is caused by aging, menopause, or another health condition. Many people, men and women alike, blame menopause for what are either normal signs of aging or the results of another medical issue or lifestyle habits. Then menopause gets a bad rap. In the following scenario, can you tell which of Ella's problems is actually caused by menopause?

Ella

Okay, so I'm menopausal. I can deal with that. The hot flashes aren't too bad, and I actually like not having periods anymore. But my skin is getting wrinkly, I'm losing my hair, and my doctor says my blood pressure's up. Even worse, when I laugh or cough, my bladder leaks a little. It's embarrassing!

Are these more symptoms of menopause? If they are, sign me up for hormone therapy—they're driving me crazy!

Because of the uncertainty of what actually caused a problem, many people—men and women alike—readily blame menopause for what are either normal signs of aging or the results of another medical issue or lifestyle habits. Then menopause gets a bad rap.

Signposts on the Road

Our bodies send us reminders that they need attention, particularly if we're not taking good care of ourselves. If you slack off on regular exercise and healthy eating, your cholesterol and blood pressure will rise. If you don't get enough sleep or do enough stretching, you might be irritable or feel stiff. Maybe you're unable to think of the right word or remember where you put your keys because you're tired, distracted, or trying to do too many things. These signals often hit at the same time as menopause cues, such as hot flashes, mood swings, and skin changes.

But the reasons for the signals aren't always clear. Are they age related, or are they due to menopause? It's like a traffic jam: you're not sure whether you're sitting in bumper-to-bumper traffic because of an accident up ahead or simply because everyone left work at the same time.

Of course, our bodies don't always produce changes in a way that lets us deal with one problem at a time. This explains why so many women come into my office feeling betrayed by their bodies and asking such questions as these:

- Why did I put on ten pounds when I'm just as active as I was at 25?

- I haven't changed my eating habits, so why is my cholesterol suddenly so high?

- How can I control my blood pressure when my job is so stressful?

Teasing out symptoms of menopause from aging or other conditions is not always easy. I usually start by explaining to my patients what I call the "target zones," the places where age and menopause often conflict.

Before we can treat a conflict in a target zone, we need to find out what started the war, a sometimes complicated process.

Your Target Zones: Where Age and Hormones Intersect

Several areas in the body are affected by both aging and hormonal influences, so let us examine those, as well as effects from both aging and hormone loss alone.

Eyes

Age. There's a reason you remember your grandma peering through bifocals as she read the newspaper. And you've probably noticed that your glasses prescription doesn't *improve* with every visit to the eye doctor.

The explanation is purely scientific. The lens of the eye, located behind the cornea, loses its flexibility as we age, causing a decrease in our ability to focus on small print. Because of this, even those of us who started out with twenty-twenty vision will eventually be reaching for reading glasses.

Hormones. The cornea reacts to rapid shifts in hormones. These can occur while you're pregnant or using birth control pills, other hormonal contraception, or HT. The diameter of the cornea changes with hormonal fluctuations; changes in the shape of the lens depend on how much water it contains. This can affect your vision. It is best to avoid having laser eye surgery or getting fitted for contacts when your cornea may be under the influence of hormone fluctuations.

Skin

Age. The sun is the main offender when it comes to skin damage. Over time, sunburns, visits to the tanning bed, and disregard for sun blockers contribute to solar aging, resulting in the loss of elasticity and the appearance of wrinkles. Compare your face to less exposed areas of your body, where you'll find smoother skin. You know what I'm talking about!

Toxins such as cigarette smoke can also age skin significantly. In other cases, simple genetics and darker skin explain why some women look younger than their chronological age.

Hormones. Consider a pregnant woman whose skin is glowing. Hormone levels are high at this point in her life.

With the dramatic loss of hormones comes loss of collagen, the connective tissue in the skin responsible for its elasticity and resilience (collagen gives skin that "plumpness"). Some women experience as much as a 30 to 40 percent loss of collagen within five years of menopause.

Research shows that estrogen clearly helps maintain collagen levels, and women who choose to take estrogen therapy may report less aging in their skin. Of course, this is not the sole reason to begin hormone therapy. (We'll talk about this more in chapter 5.)

Hair

Age. At least 40 to 50 percent of women lose some hair or notice thinning as they age.

Hormones. Hair loss can worsen with lack of estrogen, as well as the increased sensitivity to testosterone based on lowered relative estrogen levels you experience in menopause. Skin, hair, and nails are all affected by hormones, nutrition, and genetics.

Heart Rate

Age. You can pump your legs just as fast on that walk today as you did when you were 22 years old, but your heart rate won't climb as quickly or as high as it did then. It's an ironic rite of passage that we have to work harder to increase our heart rate when we get older. And with age, our maximum heart rate decreases.

Hormones. Estrogen affects women's electrical cardiac rhythms. Women tend to have a longer QT interval on their EKG (electrocardiogram) tracings and are more predisposed to "falsely abnormal" EKG stress tests. (The QT interval is a measure of the time between the start of one wave, the Q wave, and the end of another—the T wave—in the heart's electrical cycle.) Most important, women are more likely than men to experience adverse disturbance to their heart rhythms when they take certain medications. In fact, most medications that have been taken off the market because of heart arrhythmia problems were disproportionately problematic for women.

Cholesterol

Age. Cholesterol may or may not increase with age; this is mostly determined by genetics, diet, and lifestyle. But if your weight and diet change as you gain in years, your cholesterol will almost certainly rise.

Hormones. Estrogen helps improve the cardio-protective, "good" HDL cholesterol and keep the "bad" LDL cholesterol in check. Loss of estrogen in some women (with all other things held constant, such as diet and weight) may cause cholesterol levels to worsen.

If a woman gains the infamous "menopausal 15" on top of the "freshman 15" of her college days, as well as "mommy weight" she might have acquired after having babies, she can easily slip into elevated cholesterol, elevated blood pressure, and even diabetes almost overnight.

Metabolism

Age. By midlife, few of us can get away with drive-through dinners or late-night eating without tipping the scale. As we celebrate more birthdays, metabolism naturally slows. Simultaneously, we lose muscle mass, and since muscle helps burn calories, our bodies must work harder for us to afford any extra portions or desserts.

Hormones. Whether you're naturally menopausal or your ovaries were removed through hysterectomy, you are likely to notice an accelerated loss of muscle mass. The way to combat this is with

Is It True That Hormone Therapy Will Make Me Gain Weight?

This is a common myth. No, you will not gain weight by taking hormones. In fact, women who take hormones are less likely to gain weight than those who are not on HT because they better maintain lean muscle mass. Some women on hormones even lose weight (usually only a pound or two—this is no reason to begin HT).

Women who gain weight on hormones are neglecting proper nutrition and exercise, unless they are reporting water weight gain. Higher doses of estrogen can promote salt and water retention in some women, which can be easily managed by restricting salt intake, reducing the estrogen dose, or occasionally using diuretics. If you maintain a healthy lifestyle and choose to take hormones, you should not notice weight fluctuation.

weight-bearing exercise such as strength training, which will help build muscle mass. You can do this. I know many women in midlife and beyond who are stronger and in better shape than some 20 or 30 year olds.

Bone Mass

Age. We rapidly make deposits in our bone bank during adolescence, which explains why it's so important for our teenage daughters (and sons) to drink milk rather than switch to soft drinks. We continue to build bone mass until age 30, when it peaks. From then on, we generally cannot accrue bone—we only lose it.

Hormones. At least half of all women will lose bone at a rapid pace after entering menopause. Much of this has to do with family history.

Also, if you weigh less than 127 pounds and/or smoke cigarettes, you're more likely to be diagnosed with low bone mass (osteopenia), a condition in which there is decreased bone-mineral density. This is generally a precursor to osteoporosis, a more serious condition in which bones become brittle and can possibly break. Most women who suffer a broken bone actually have osteopenia, but both require treatment or at least preventive therapy. See chapter 12 for more on bone health.

Are There Any Conditions Solely Related to Aging?

Of course, some health conditions are simply age related. Just as certain parts of a car wear out or need a tune-up after a while, certain body functions sputter when we hit midlife, and our personal "maintenance lights" switch on. Follwing are some changes to watch for:

Kidney Function. Think of the kidneys as your internal cleaning crew. After years of working overtime, especially if they're stressed by the symptoms of high blood pressure or diabetes, they get tired. Starting at age 30, there's a slow decline in kidney function and how our bodies remove raw waste. Most of us don't recognize any problems because enough of the "cleaning crew" is still doing its job.

Bone Loss. You can get calcium from foods—soy and dairy products; greens like spinach and broccoli; and even fortified breads, cereals, and orange juice. But unless you drink a glass of skim milk three times a day, chances are slim that you're meeting all your calcium needs through food.

To maintain their current bone mass, women age 30 and older need at least 1,200 milligrams (mg) of calcium daily, in addition to at least 1,000 international units (IU) of vitamin D each day (the vitamin D is particularly important if they avoid sun exposure and do not drink cod liver oil). Women over age 55 who do not take estrogen experience a reduction in the intestines' ability to absorb calcium and need to ingest 1,500 mg of calcium daily and at least 1,000 IU to 2,000 IU of vitamin D3 (cholecaliferol).

Some women who get the proper amounts of calcium and vitamin D still lose bone rapidly after menopause. These women may have a family history of osteoporosis, hip fracture, dowager's hump, or height loss. Having low body fat or a current or past eating disorder also can reduce your bone mass. Diet and exercise regimes can be a factor. Both a history of kidney stones (some women excrete too much calcium in their urine) and a history of wheat/gluten intolerance (celiac disease), which reduces the body's ability to absorb enough vitamin D and iron, can affect bone loss. Smoking cigarettes is another harmful factor. Of course, if you smoke, quit. Now. And talk to your doctor about devising an anti-osteoporosis program that takes all your personal risk factors into account. (For more on preventing bone loss, see chapter 12.)

• • • *Fast Fact* • • •

When considering how you take your calcium, keep in
mind that your body can only absorb 500 mg of calcium
at a time. Like a sponge that gets saturated and can't
take in any more liquid, your gut gets "saturated" with
calcium. If you take 1,200 mg all at once, anything
more than 500 mg will not be absorbed.

• • •

Blood Pressure. Rising blood pressure is something that men and
women have in common as they age. Blood pressure increases in
many adults, particularly between the ages 35 to 55, and may continue to rise thereafter.

As mentioned earlier, for women, blood pressure should be
115/75 or less.

Bladder Control. Losing control over your bladder is no laughing matter, but laughing—as well as sneezing, coughing, and
jumping—can trigger accidents in many women as they get
older. The medical term for leaking urine is "urinary incontinence." "Stress incontinence" occurs involuntarily with laughing,

Red Flag

Involuntarily leaking urine is *not* a part of normal aging and not
a normal part of menopause, either. If you are wearing a pad
or liner because of leakage, or you are afraid to jump on the
trampoline with grandchildren or to see a funny movie for fear of
bladder leakage, please see your physician or a urogynecologist.
If you are contemplating surgery, see a surgeon who specializes
in leaky bladders.

jumping, or coughing. "Urge incontinence" results from the type of overactive bladder that wants to empty as soon as you feel the slightest urge—it's as if your bladder has a mind of its own. Some women have "mixed" incontinence, which includes both stress and urge leakage.

"Stress urinary incontinence," or SUI, is usually related to lack of support of the bladder neck and is worsened with weight gain, constipation, childbearing, chronic cough, and enlarged uterus (women on high doses of HT may have a larger/heavier uterus and might notice worsening of this type of leakage). If you have SUI, you might try inserting a supersized tampon into the vagina to see if this reduces leakage—if this does help, it generally means your bladder neck needs additional support. Many effective therapies provide relief from this condition, including collagen injections, exercise, biofeedback, and even surgical repair procedures.

If you have "urge incontinence" or "overactive bladder" (OAB), you need to see a doctor to have a urinalysis (to exclude infection or bladder abnormality) and a "postvoid residual" bladder scan to see if there is any leftover urine left in your bladder after emptying it (less than 50 cc is normal). If both of these tests are normal, you should be advised to avoid bladder irritants such as caffeine, alcohol, acidic drinks, carbonated beverages, artificial sweeteners, and spicy foods. Bladder retraining and "timed voiding," as well as keeping a journal of your food and drink intake, and the number of times you urinate, will be helpful for you and your doctor. There are many prescription OAB medications such as the oral forms of DETROL LA (tolterodine tartrate), ENABLEX (darifenacin), SANCTURA XR (trospium), VESIcare (solifenacin succinate), or the oral or patch form of DITROPAN XL (oxybutynin chloride). These OAB medicines should not be taken if you have acute angle glaucoma. They may cause constipation or dry mouth. If one agent doesn't work or causes dry mouth, then I encourage patients to try another, as some women respond better to one agent than another.

Kegel Exercises

All women should do Kegel exercises (20 to 25 repetitions) every morning. Do them standing up, maybe while you brush your teeth. Most of us never forget to brush our teeth, but many women forget about their pelvic muscles. If you are unable to do Kegel exercises or are unsure how to do them, ask your physician to instruct you while performing a pelvic exam; the examiner can detect pelvic tone and pelvic support.

Some women are completely unable to contract these muscles properly and need to be referred to a physical therapist who specializes in the pelvic floor. Muscle rehabilitation and pelvic biofeedback can be used to improve problems with muscle tone.

For very mild cases of mixed incontinence in women with atrophic, thin vaginas, I have found the Estring (Estradiol Vaginal Ring) to be very helpful when combined with pelvic exercises (Kegels) and bladder behavioral retraining.

Lack of local estrogen can affect both the vagina and the base of the bladder, and this may be one factor in making the bladder more irritable and more susceptible to infection. Conversely, systemic HT may increase the size and weight of the uterus, which may put some pressure on the bladder.

Bladder control relates to many factors—muscles, nerves, the bladder lining, hormones, and the supporting muscles and structures—and we've just discussed the fact that we lose muscle mass as we age. The pelvic muscle, called the levator ani, supports the bladder, uterus, top of the vagina, and rectum. It is the muscle you consciously contract to stop the flow of urine, stool, or gas, and that involuntarily contracts during sexual climax. These same pelvic muscles can be damaged during pregnancy and childbirth and can be strained with weight gain. If you don't exercise the pelvic muscles, you can lose strength, which is why I always recommend that women practice Kegel exercises.

Is It Age, or Is It Menopause?

When I can't separate menopausal symptoms from age-related changes in my patients, the best course of action is to use a low dose of hormone therapy to see whether that resolves the problem. If it does, we know that the symptom was menopause related.

For example, if I prescribe hormones and my patient finds that her hot flashes are reduced, and she is sleeping better and feels less anxious, then her symptoms were probably menopausal. We can adjust her HT as necessary. If her symptoms are not resolved, we know there's another cause that has yet to be found and treated.

As for Ella (whose situation was described at the beginning of this chapter), I explained to her that her skin and hair problems were most likely related to menopause, but the rise in her blood pressure and the embarrassing bladder leaks were probably related to lifestyle, genetics, and age.

After I offered some tips for dealing with skin and hair problems at midlife (which I'll go into in chapter 5), she decided to try some alternatives to HT and see whether her symptoms improved.

We decided to work together on keeping her blood pressure within a healthy range, and after a urinalysis, pelvic exam, and bladder scan to see whether there was residual urine in the bladder after voiding, I referred her to a urogynecologist (a surgeon who specializes in both the medical and surgical treatment of bladder leakage in women).

"Brain Fog" and Other Memory Problems

Memory difficulty frequently rounds out a suite of other menopause symptoms, and women who have hot flashes and sleep loss often say that they struggle to find words or just don't feel like themselves. They aren't absent-minded professors; their thinking just isn't sharp. Many describe it as "brain fog." If this sounds familiar, you're not losing your mind. Most likely, you're not developing Alzheimer's disease either.

Sandra

It's like a fog—a haze that settles into my brain like a cloud. I'll be explaining to my husband some event that happened during the day, and I'll blank out on a simple word. "I just dropped Michelle off at day camp, and her . . ."

"Teacher," my husband will fill in, nodding at me to tell him what happened next.

It's so embarrassing. Nowadays I feel as if people must think "Sandra's losing her mind." Well, some days it does feel that way, but I'm sure every working mother of two forgets where she is or what she has to do sometimes—we have so many places to be and so many things to do!

But I'm getting worried. My mother had Alzheimer's. Come to think of it, nearly every woman in her nursing home had that blank, far-off stare. It scares me that I may be following in her footsteps.

Perhaps you can relate your brain fog to the same hazy feeling that some postpartum women experience after delivering. I remember that after I had my first child, I couldn't even write thank-you notes for baby gifts. I couldn't spell simple words like *where* and *when*. Duh!

That's because hormones fluctuate rapidly after giving birth. The sudden inability to recall simple facts or information, like the spelling of everyday words, happens when estrogen levels drop extremely low.

You see, estrogen is brain food. Dipping levels of estrogen, whether from having a baby or going into menopause, affect brain function. Throw sleep deprivation and hot flashes into the mix, along with other medical changes that occur in midlife, and you can see why your brain is not functioning on all cylinders. It's normal, though frustrating. Please don't let it scare you.

How Do I Know It Isn't Alzheimer's?

Here are some facts to ease your concerns if you struggle with memory "blips," as I call them.

- People who have Alzheimer's are not so aware of their condition that they can recognize it and tell the doctors.

- Many times, the first symptom of Alzheimer's is forgetting how to perform activities, such as driving home from the store or carrying out simple motor functions (this is called "apraxia"), not simply fumbling for the right words.

- Rarely do adults in their 40s and 50s have Alzheimer's. Generally speaking, people who suffer from this disease are much older.

- The good news is that the "brain fog" that accompanies midlife can be treated, and further memory loss may be prevented by stimulating your brain on a regular basis.

Can Hormone Therapy Help Relieve My Memory Problems?

Sometimes, HT can be used to sharpen memory. Observational data from a study in Cache County, Utah, suggest that hormone therapy prescribed during menopause might protect the brain from memory loss, but the researchers are careful to note that observational data are not grounds for prescribing estrogen for this express purpose.

In the study, women who began hormone therapy in menopause and continued it for ten years developed Alzheimer's at half the rate of women who never took hormones.

We can deduce from this research that taking HT for a few years around the time of menopause may be beneficial in preventing memory loss. (Of course, as with any prescription drug, every woman's case is unique and must be examined thoroughly.)

This information isn't definitive, but it is provocative. I wouldn't tell a woman to take hormone therapy to reduce the risk of Alzheimer's disease down the road, but if she suffers from memory complaints around the time of menopause and I can rule out thyroid disease, vitamin B_{12} deficiency, and depression as possible causes, I would definitely recommend a trial of HT for a short time and then reassess her status. If she responds, I'd keep her on therapy and re-evaluate her annually. If she shows no response, I'd refer her to a neurologist for more detailed testing.

What Else Can I Do to Keep My Memory Sharp?

Through a fascinating study of aging nuns called, appropriately enough, the Nun Study, we're learning more about what factors in early, mid-, and late life increase the risk of Alzheimer's.

Funded by the National Institute on Aging, this longitudinal study began in 1986 as a pilot study on aging and disability, using data collected from the order School Sisters of Notre Dame living in Mankato, Minnesota. In 1990, the study was expanded to include School Sisters living in other U.S. regions.

The 678 participants were 75 to 103 years old, with an average age of 85. The group represented a wide range of health and level of function. More than 85 percent of the women had been teachers. All agreed before joining the study to donate their brains to the research effort after death.

Results showed that some nuns in the study who lived to be more than 100 years old still retained their intellectual faculties, even though there was evidence of Alzheimer's plaques in their brains. The researchers discovered that these nuns had stayed quite engaged mentally. They learned new languages. They wrote in journals. They participated in mental workouts and exercised their brains, and they stayed sharp right up to their last days.

This link between mental activity and decreased chance of Alzheimer's is a very important finding, with implications far beyond the convent. In my opinion, it certainly points to a definite role for brain exercise.

Brain Boosters. If your job is left-brained, relax by performing right-brained activities. For example, if you work as an accountant, in your spare time, do something physical or creative. Go for a vigorous walk, read a novel, take up ballroom dancing.

However, if your job is right-brained and creative—say you're a writer—then you want to stretch your analytical left brain. Play chess or Monopoly or do crossword puzzles.

Now, we know that even if they're not in paid employment, all women work, so the trick is for all women to engage and challenge both the right and the left sides of the brain, whether they work in an office or at home with their children. Try learning a foreign language or maybe how to tango. Read and write; try journaling about happy things that you experience day to day. This will help both your brain health and your mood.

Enough of the Bad News

Please highlight this part of the chapter. Read it out loud and make it your anthem.

Midlife is not the beginning of the end. It's the beginning of the best years, which are still to come. We mature and change, but many women feel most comfortable in their skin during midlife and beyond. You've acquired wisdom and experience, and perhaps more confidence. Your perspective and skills are sharpened.

Perhaps some nagging symptoms or body changes have inspired you to clean up your act and take care of your body, and as a result, you're feeling better than ever.

Remember: *You* are in control. There are solutions and options for you as your body experiences this new phase in life. And only the very rare woman says that she regrets the absence of her monthly period.

It's never too late to adopt healthy habits for the rest of our lives. Exercising really does counteract aging. Midlife can be the perfect time to reinvent yourself, learn a new skill, renew old friendships, and begin some new ones, as well as make new spiritual and/or career connections.

The more you know, the more you can control your vitality and health.

Chapter 4

Maintaining Mood at Midlife

For many women, midlife is a welcome lifestyle change. Newly emptied nests produce more free time and a relaxing of responsibilities. We can enjoy hobbies we set aside during our child-raising years, or we might choose to travel, advance our careers, or explore new ventures. With such newfound freedoms, we are likely to feel happy and on an "even keel."

On the other hand, some women face increased stresses on the home front during midlife. As the humorist Erma Bombeck wrote, "I'm trying very hard to understand this generation. They have adjusted the timetable for childbearing so that menopause and teaching a 16-year-old how to drive a car will occur in the same week."

Often, women are called on to care for their aging, sometimes ailing parents. This responsibility can take its toll on your time, emotional balance, sleep, and certainly mood.

In midlife, you may also be dealing with divorce, career-related problems, or the death of someone you love. All these will naturally affect your mood and may leave you feeling depressed.

Another take on depression at the time of menopause suggests that hormone-related physical changes mar a woman's self-image and leave her feeling a little down. With drier skin and thinning vaginal walls, she doesn't look or feel as beautiful and sexy as she did five years earlier. And looking into the mirror only to see thinning hair and dull skin doesn't do much for one's self-esteem.

Although this kind of depression may seem based on superficialities, most women can attest to that "look good, feel good" motto. When we're happy about our health and appearance, we have a better outlook on life.

Depression and Menopause

Menopause is not a major risk for clinical depression. However, the hormone changes that occur at this point in a woman's life can influence the neurotransmitters in the brain—serotonin, dopamine, and norepinephrine—that regulate brain function. This trio of neurotransmitters sends messages to various parts of the brain responsible for functions such as sleep, appetite, mood, sexual interest, and sense of well-being.

Estrogen may stimulate the brain and boost serotonin, while progesterone may reduce serotonin. Rapid fluxes in hormone levels can throw some women out of synch. Considering this, it's not far-fetched to say that menopause can be the breaking point that throws a woman's mood into a tailspin, particularly if her neurotransmitters are already running on empty. Some of my patients have referred to this experience as "reverse puberty."

The fact is that one in three women will be diagnosed with major depression at some point in her life. This frequently coincides with menopause, particularly if the perimenopausal transition is especially long or difficult.

Let's take a look at Janet's situation.

Janet
I'm looking in the mirror, trying to put on a happy face, talking myself into shaking off the down-and-out attitude I've been waking up with for weeks.

With hot flashes waking me every hour at night, things just don't seem manageable in the morning. My teenage son requires more attention than he did when he was in elementary school, and I don't want to let him see his mom fall apart. And after her surgery for hip fracture, my own mother needs me more than ever.

My husband and I enjoy each other's company, but I can't seem to take pleasure in the same things we used to look forward to doing together—dancing, cooking with friends, hiking. I just go through the motions.

I've never been such a drag! And I can't think of any time I ever felt this down. Even PMS was never a problem for me. I've always been stable, enjoying life, not letting the inevitable stresses get to me.

I stopped getting my period five months ago, so I must be going into menopause. Lately those cartoons poking fun at menopausal women who flip out seem like a disturbing portrait of me! Who is this lady in the mirror this morning, and how do I get my self back?

• • • **Fast Fact** • • •

Women are two to three times more likely than men
to suffer from depression.

• • •

For women who did not experience any form of depression after delivering children, during PMS, or while caring for young children (all times when depression is common in women), feeling blue at midlife, as Janet's case indicates, vividly contradicts what they have previously experienced during times of hormone flucuations. Menopause can aggravate existing depression, and women who are not already depressed but begin suffering from menopausal side effects, such as hot flashes, are also likely to suffer from an episode of depression.

Which Comes First, Menopause or Depression?

Answering this question is not easy. Today, research suggests that during the time a woman is making the transition into menopause, she is at risk for depression, particularly if that transition is tumultuous.

I see proof of this in my office every week. Women with no family history or personal experience of depression suddenly feel helplessly down and out. They've been healthy, medically stable, and free of major stressors. Then *bam!* Menopause hits. They're having mood swings, precipitated in part by lack of sleep as hot flashes keep waking them up. They get up in the morning feeling irritable. They're uncomfortable. And they become concerned about their higher blood pressure, rising cholesterol, and stubborn weight gain. Everything seems to collide at one point—midlife.

We can't pinpoint exactly what makes hormones and neurotransmitters interact differently in menopausal women who suffer

Depression Is Different in Women and Men

For women, depression may occur earlier, last longer, and be more likely to recur. Women are more sensitive to life events and changes of seasons, both of which can trigger depression. Depression in women is more often associated with anxiety disorders, especially panic and phobic symptoms, and eating disorders. Women are more likely to experience guilty feelings and attempt suicide when depressed; however, men are more likely actually to commit suicide.

from depression, compared with menopausal women who don't get depressed.

The key is to understand that there are various types of depression, to recognize the signs, and most important, to remember that depression is a treatable condition, not a sign of weakness or something you should be ashamed about. You can do something about it and feel better.

Is Feeling "Blue" a Sign of Depression?

Feeling sad or just "not yourself" is not depression. It's normal to feel dejected when your boss gives you only a satisfactory review or you notice that your skinny jeans are hugging your curves a bit too closely. It's also normal to respond deeply to the death of a loved one and feel quite sad for weeks or even months. These responses are unlike major depression, also called "clinical depression," which is a bona fide medical condition involving imbalances in brain chemistry.

Consider Lila.

Lila

When my father died, my world collapsed. He was my mentor, and I took over his business when he retired. I never imagined what life would be like without his support and love. I mourned for months, and every year, joyous occasions like cutting down the family Christmas tree were bittersweet. But I worked through those feelings.

My sadness then was nothing like the cloud that hovered over my days during menopause. I felt desperate and helpless. The persistent gloom and unhappiness felt like a lead vest that dragged down my every activity.

What Lila experienced after the loss of her father was normal sadness. But later, during menopause, she went into depression.

Are You Depressed? A Quick Quiz

No two women will experience exactly the same symptoms of depression, but there are questions you can ask yourself to determine whether your mood is something beyond just feeling blue.

If you suspect clinical depression, discuss your concerns with a physician. If you answer yes to any of these questions, she will want to explore your condition further:

- Have you lost interest in hobbies or activities that you used to enjoy?
- Do you have trouble falling or staying asleep? Are you tired all the time, regardless of how much you sleep?
- Do you feel resentful or angry? Do you have outbursts of complaints or shouting?
- Have you lost interest in sex?
- Do you feel worthless, unattractive, or guilty for no reason?
- Do you struggle to concentrate? Are your thoughts muddy or foggy?
- Do you have slow body movements or speech?
- Do you brood or experience delusions or fears? Do you often feel anxious?
- Have you had periods of mania, mood elevation, and/or inability to sleep?
- Have you considered suicide?

The level and severity of similar emotions is markedly different in depression. Just as feeling blue should not cause you undue worry, drastic plunges in feelings of self-worth, interest in activities and friends, and general happiness should not be brushed aside.

What Are the Symptoms of a Mood Disorder?

Symptoms of various mood disorders can mimic those of menopause. Anxiety, sweats, heart palpitations—is this a panic attack or menopause? We're edgy one minute, forgetful the next. Is this something more than naturally occurring menopause? ADHD, perhaps?

When teasing out symptoms of depression from menopause, we run into the whodunit of women's health. Searching for the culprit causing one's symptoms often results in a lineup of health problems, and usually more than one "suspect," or diagnosis, is guilty.

Fortunately, we can distinguish serious mood disorders from basic menopause symptoms during a thorough examination and interview, and we can treat such disorders while easing menopausal side effects.

First, we must understand the indications for major depression and other disorders that affect mood and/or behavior, including panic disorder, bipolar disorder, obsessive-compulsive disorder, and ADHD.

Major Depression. Major depression is characterized by general feelings of sadness or worthlessness. Those who suffer from major depression answer yes to most if not all of the questions listed on page 62.

Here are some symptoms of depression:

Emotional: Complete loss of pleasure in things that were once enjoyable, trouble sleeping or eating, lack of interest in sex, and suicidal thoughts.

Physical: Weight gain or loss and insomnia or tiredness despite getting adequate sleep.

Panic Disorder. Of all the mood disorders associated with meno-pause, panic disorder is one of the most vexing. Its intense physical symptoms may drive women to visit many different types of physicians, as Kathy did (page X), in their search for relief.

Panic disorder involves more than an occasional bout of anxiety. Women with panic disorder may have frequent panic attacks, often worry for more than a month about having another one, and change their behavior in the hope of avoiding another attack. They may go to the emergency room only to be told that they're fine.

Panic disorder is often accompanied by depression and mood swings. It affects 3 to 4 percent of women, regardless of their menstrual status.

A woman with panic disorder may see all kinds of different specialists over a period of years without receiving a correct diagnosis.

Heart palpitations may lead her to a cardiologist, who, after testing, will report "normal" results. A neurologist will check her when she complains of dizziness or headaches. No diagnosis there. Anxiety, sweating, and palpitations mirror many symptoms of menopause, so she may again be told that she's "only going through the change."

When panic disorder and menopause intersect, a woman can feel as if her world is exploding. Many times menopause treatment, medication for panic disorder, and supportive therapy all have to be started at once. Kathy received this trio of treatments and within a few months was back to her usual self. Within a year she was off all therapy, and she continues to do very well.

The symptoms of panic disorder include these:

Emotional: Sudden, intense feeling of doom or apprehension.

Physical: Heart palpitations, shortness of breath, dizziness, weakness, sweating, nausea, and tingling sensations.

Bipolar Disorder (Manic-Depressive). As the name of the disorder suggests, women with bipolar disorder experience periods of mania, then deep depression. Experiencing extremely high and extremely low moods, those who suffer from this disorder can feel elated, irritable, and paranoid all within a matter of minutes. The world is full of possibilities one day; the next, it's doom and gloom.

If you're bipolar, you're probably hyperactive and may talk quickly and loudly, switching rapidly from one topic to the next, or maybe you have periods when you don't sleep. Perhaps your first episode included severe postpartum depression.

People with bipolar illness may get worse if they're treated only with standard antidepressants such as SSRIs (selective serotonin reuptake inhibitors), which may trigger a manic episode. Women with bipolar illness need to be treated with medications such as lithium (a naturally occurring element in the periodic table) or LAMICTAL (lamotrigine) or DEPAKOTE (valproic acid), which are anticonvulsants that help stabilize the brain. Other medicines like ABILIFY (aripiprazole), an atypical antipsychotic that works as a mood stabilizer and is FDA approved to treat bipolar illness, may be needed.

Following are symptoms of mania in bipolar disorder:

Emotional: Extremely high spirits; delusions about capabilities; excessive, risky behavior; overly euphoric mood; racing thoughts; anger; inability to sleep.

Physical: Forceful, rapid speech; less need for sleep; rebellious behavior.

Obsessive-Compulsive Disorder (OCD). OCD involves obsessive and distressing involuntary ideas, fears, or impulses that recur. The anxiety that follows such ideas sometimes drives the patient to perform certain routines (compulsions) to find calm or stability. Examples include hand washing, counting, checking, hoarding, repeating, cleaning, and endlessly rearranging objects. People with OCD feel as if performing such rituals is a life-or-death necessity.

Most people with OCD know that this behavior is not reasonable. In fact, they often become depressed because they recognize the problems that the disorder is causing in their lives.

Symptoms of obsessive-compulsive disorder include the following:

Emotional: Anxiety, distress, fear.

Physical: Repetitive and ritualistic behavior.

Attention Deficit Hyperactivity Disorder (ADHD). Anna had been seeing me for one year for treatment of her severe menopausal symptoms. The last time she was in my office, she said, "I think I have ADHD."

I was surprised at first. "Why now? What makes you think that?" I asked. She told me that her son had been diagnosed a few months before, and she recognized his symptoms in her own behavior.

It's not surprising that many adults are diagnosed with ADHD after their children are found to have the disorder. Parents tend to think of ADHD as a social and academic inhibitor for children and adolescents. But as they learn what behaviors are associated with ADHD—for example, being easily distracted, having trouble sitting still, being impulsive—they wonder if their own lack of concentration and restless behavior might represent the same condition.

The following symptoms can be signs of either menopause or ADHD. If we decide to try a low dose of hormone therapy and the symptoms don't improve, we consider whether or not the problem may be ADHD related.

Here are some symptoms of attention deficit hyperactivity disorder:

Emotional: Problems prioritizing tasks, feeling of being "flaky" or "scatterbrained," easily distracted.

Physical: Inability to meet work deadlines or keep appointments, frequent forgetfulness, a hectic and disorganized appearance.

What Do I Do If My Mood or Personality Alters During Menopause?

Noticing mood shifts or feeling not quite yourself is perfectly normal during perimenopause and menopause.

Depending on how severe your menopause symptoms are, you may become more vulnerable to mood swings because of lack of sleep or physical discomfort. Your energy reserves are low, decreasing your tolerance for stressors. You feel absentminded and forgetful. You break down when your daughter comes home from school with a poor report card. You snap at your housebound mother, whom you love dearly, when she asks you to pick up milk at the store. If you've never been particularly moody, such feelings may especially spark concern.

In these cases, the root of a woman's emotional frailty might be menopause, and treating symptoms with lifestyle changes (diet and exercise) or hormone therapy, if appropriate, will level out the hormone imbalance that is agitating her mood.

On the other hand, if the descriptions in this chapter really seem to apply to you, you'll want to dig deeper. Gather your family history (remember that pink folder you're keeping?) and talk with your doctor. She'll want to conduct medical tests to rule out underactive thyroid, anemia, diabetes, adrenal insufficiency, or hepatitis, all of which can cause depression and, fortunately, can be treated.

During your appointment, you should tell your doctor about any and all medications you take, including vitamins, herbal remedies, diet supplements, and recreational drugs, in case they're contributing to your problems.

What Kind of Treatment Options Exist for Mood Disorders During Menopause?

During perimenopause and menopause, depression and other mood disorders are treated in much the same way they are at other times. Antidepressants and cognitive and behavioral therapy can all help. Hormones may also help improve mood.

So what's the solution—hormone therapy, antidepressants, or a combination? Here are a few different scenarios.

You Feel Depressed, "Not Yourself," and Are Not Being Treated with Hormone Therapy. Hormone therapy can help reduce hot flashes and night sweats, thereby restoring sleep, which in turn improves mood. Independent of its effects on hot flashes, HT may still improve mood.

Hormone therapy protects the vaginal area against thinning and dryness, making sex more enjoyable. Hormones also protect skin from collagen loss, so women may feel better about the way their skin looks.

In general, many women who take HT do not suffer from the irritable side effects of menopause that can drag down their mood and reduce their tolerance for stress.

You Take a Low Dose of Estrogen but Still Feel Moody and Blue All the Time. When a woman taking hormone therapy still feels depressed, I examine her dosage. The current trend is to prescribe lower doses of hormones for shorter periods. Logically, this may reduce side effects and risks because women are taking less medication. That's a good thing. However, we may also be undertreating a woman's condition, which is not such a good thing.

The less-is-more theory doesn't apply to every woman's health needs. She may feel better and less depressed if her HT prescription is increased. I sometimes choose to do this before using mood medicines. I try my best to listen to my patients since they are often able to tell me whether they need more or less HT, more antidepressant, or a different medication altogether.

Your Doctor Recently Increased Your Hormone Therapy Dosage, but You Still Feel Anxious, Panicky, or Downright Depressed. If a woman is receiving an adequate level of hormone therapy and still feels depressed, I consider antidepressant therapy. We may need to treat menopause and depression concurrently to achieve the best results.

If I suspect major clinical depression, regardless of the woman's hormone status, I recommend treatment with an antidepressant medicine and/or cognitive behavioral therapy. Both are effective ways to treat depression and when combined give the best results.

What Antidepressants Are Best for Use by Menopausal Women?

I prescribe low doses of antidepressant at first to test a woman's response to the medication. If the response is good and she starts to feel less moody, I will continue the treatment for at least six to nine months after the point that she feels like her usual self. Standard antidepressants, such as the SSRIs and the SNRIs (serotonin-norepinephrine reuptake inhibitors), are not addictive and do not change your personality.

SSRIs. There are many types of antidepressants, including the SSRIs Prozac (fluoxetine) and Zoloft (sertraline), and these are available in generic formulations.

- SARAFEM (fluoxetine): The first SSRI to be FDA approved to treat severe PMS.

- LEXAPRO (escitalopram): The active ingredient of a previously popular antidepressant, Celexa (citalopram), LEXAPRO does not interfere with hormone levels or many other medications metabolized in the liver. I prescribe this agent for women with severe PMS or generalized anxiety disorder, as well as for women suffering with major depression or panic disorder. It comes in a liquid formulation whose dose can be gradually adjusted in sensitive patients.

- Paxil (paroxetine): I don't tend to prescribe Paxil as it is associated with constipation and weight gain and can reduce Tamoxifen (a drug used to treat as well as prevent breast cancer) levels in some patients.

- Prozac (fluoxetine): A commonly used antidepressant with a long half-life

- Zoloft (sertraline): A commonly used antidepressant with a short half-life

SNRIs. The SNRIs (serotonin-norepinephrine reuptake inhibitors), like the SSRIs are not addictive and do not change your personality. They affect the norepinephrine neurotransmitter system as well as the serotonin.

- CYMBALTA (duloxetine): This drug may help reduce stress urinary incontinence, but it's important to monitor liver function while taking it.

- EFFEXOR XR (venlafaxine): I frequently prescribe this drug for women with hot flashes.

- PRISTIQ (desvenlafaxine): I also may prescribe this drug for women with hot flashes, as it is the active ingredient of

Bone Density and Antidepressants

Women on long-term antidepressants may have a lower bone density—in part from having depression and/or from the SSRI effect on the bone. Further research is needed in this area; however, if you have depression, you should be treated, and your bones can always be periodically monitored with bone density tests. Exercise is good for both your bones and your mood.

EFFEXOR XR (venlafaxine) and is currently FDA approved to treat depression.

- WELLBUTRIN XL (bupropion): I prescribe WELL-BUTRIN XL for women who do not have anxiety, seizure disorder, or eating disorder and who suffer from depression and/or fatigue and low motivation. WELLBUTRIN XL is also good for women currently taking SSRIs who are suffering from sexual side effects (such as a delayed ability to climax), which some SSRIs—especially at higher doses—are known to produce. WELLBUTRIN XL is known for its lack of associated weight gain and sexual side effects.

• • • *Fast Fact* • • •

Researchers are constantly testing for new and improved antidepressants that do not negatively impact sexual function. Currently, studies are being conducted on a 5-HT1A agonist called Flibanserin, which seems to be a fast-acting antidepressant that actually stimulates sex drive.

• • •

If the response is not good, I will try a different antidepressant; there are many to choose from.

What If I Am "Anti" Antidepressants?

Some women don't want to take antidepressant medication. They don't want to deal with another pill, or they're uncomfortable with the idea that they need antidepressants, reacting to a cultural stigma against mental illness that is only slowly disappearing.

Often, women grin and bear it, brushing off serious mood disorders because they see a diagnosis as a sign of weakness. Forget that! You must take care of yourself. Quite simply, you deserve it.

And if taking care of others is part of your midlife situation, you know that you must care for yourself before you can help others.

Depression is just as much a medical problem as diabetes or migraines. There's no reason to feel embarrassed or ashamed or to feel as if you should be able to conquer the condition on your own. After all, would you expect willpower alone to cure strep throat?

Can I Help Improve My Mood by Changing My Diet?

"Garbage in, garbage out" is absolutely true when it comes to food and mood. There are a number of ways you can alter your diet to improve your mood:

- Increasing omega-3 fats—the good fat found in seafood like salmon or tuna—can lift your spirits and increase your energy. I recommend at least two servings per week. If getting enough from food proves too difficult, you can also choose to take a fish oil supplement that contains omega-3s. But if women don't like fish, I prefer that they eat flaxseed, walnuts, almonds, and/or omega-3 enriched eggs because studies have shown that people who ate fish experience certain health benefits that people taking fish oil supplements do not.

- Limiting sugars may reduce the mood swings you're experiencing.

- Drink caffeine only in moderation or avoid it altogether if you don't want to feel that afternoon low when your morning java wears off.

- Avoid fast food. All those artery-clogging trans fats and related weight gain may wreak havoc on your body.

Basically, think about what you eat as fuel and consider the content of what you put into your body. When you fill up on premium, you're bound to function better.

What About Vitamin Supplements?

Even if you eat right, you still may need to ingest extra vitamins, especially vitamin D and calcium, that are critical for women in midlife. So in addition to proper diet and exercise, you may wish to explore vitamins or supplements.

You should always consult your doctor about supplements before taking them. Treat them as you would any medication. Just because you can purchase them over the counter doesn't mean they're appropriate for every woman. In fact, many over-the-counter treatments can interfere with prescription medication or even with each other, sometimes adversely affecting the consumer.

If you already take a multivitamin, be sure to read the label, do the math, and figure out how many other supplements you really need. More is not necessarily better.

B Vitamins and Mood. Many times, we are deficient in the complex of B vitamins, which help balance our mood. One reason for the deficiency is that B vitamins are destroyed by alcohol, refined sugars, nicotine, and caffeine. Also, the metabolism of some

B-complex vitamins may be altered or accelerated in women who are taking certain medications.

Relationships between B vitamins and women's bodies include the following:

- **B_1 (thiamine).** Without this vitamin, the brain rapidly runs out of energy, leading to fatigue, depression, irritability, and anxiety. Thiamine has also been used to treat menstrual cramps. I usually recommend starting with 100 mg daily.

- **B_2 (riboflavin).** This has been found to reduce migraine headaches. I usually recommend starting with 100 mg daily. Doses can go up to 400 mg.

- **B_3 (niacin).** Niacin deficiency was found to cause pellagra, which produces psychosis and dementia. Most commercial foods contain niacin, so this complication is rare. But we know that niacin deficiency can cause agitation and anxiety. Sometimes niacin is used in high doses to lower cholesterol. Unfortunately, niacin can precipitate hot flashes in some women and may irritate the liver.

- **B_5 (pantothenic acid).** This vitamin aids in hormone formation and the uptake of amino acids in the brain chemical acetylcholine, which combine to affect the brain positively.

- **B_6 (pyridoxine).** This vitamin is needed to manufacture serotonin, melatonin, and dopamine—all important for the brain. It has mild diuretic properties and has been used to treat moderate carpal tunnel syndrome. I usually recommend a trial of 50 mg daily in fatigued women. I never recommend over 100 mg daily of B_6, since high doses—such as the 200 mg that was used in the past in an attempt to treat PMS—have been associated with nerve damage.

- **B$_{12}$ (cyanocobalamin).** B$_{12}$ is important to the formation of red blood cells, as well as brain and nerve function. A B$_{12}$ deficiency may cause pernicious anemia. Or it may cause no anemia at all, instead having a negative effect on the brain and mood. A B$_{12}$ deficiency may cause mood swings, irritability, confusion, appetite loss, dizziness, heart palpitations, and neuropathy (a tingling, pins-and-needles sensation in various parts of the body). Stores of B$_{12}$ last in the body for up to five years (in contrast to folic acid, which lasts only a day or so). As they get older, many people do not absorb B$_{12}$, and people on long-term acid blockers may have reduced absorption. Individuals taking Glucophage (metformin) may also see a reduction in the B$_{12}$ levels in the body. I recommend 250 micrograms (mcg) of vitamin B$_{12}$ daily for women over age 60. Sometimes monthly B$_{12}$ shots are needed by people who have had resections (the partial removal of an organ or other body structure) of the stomach or intestines that prevent adequate B$_{12}$ absorption.

- **Folic acid.** Another form of B vitamin, folic acid aids DNA synthesis and helps produce SAMe (see below). All women of child-bearing age should ingest at least 0.4 mg of folic acid daily as this has been shown to reduce the risk of spina bifida and neural tube defects in babies. Folic acid may help with cellular repair, and I recommend 1.0 mg of folic acid daily to women who have abnormal Pap smears. (Of course, they also need to return for evaluation.)

- **SAMe.** SAMe is short for S-adenosylmethionine, a molecule the body produces from methionine, an amino acid found in protein-rich foods, and adenosine triphosphate, an energy-producing compound found in all body cells. SAMe helps form compounds in the brain, including dopamine and serotonin, that affect mood and may also improve minor joint symptoms. Though SAMe is thought to influence neurotransmitters involved in depression, its efficacy is not proven. It is important not to take SAMe if you are taking conventional antidepressants and/or if you have a history of mania or bipolar disorder.

- **Beelith.** Beelith is a combination that contains vitamin B_6 and magnesium. Vitamin B_6 is sometimes used to treat PMS, although its efficacy is debated. You may choose to take a B_{50} tablet, which has all the B complex vitamins in a 50 mg dose, and a magnesium oxide tablet, which can cost less than Beelith. That way you also get other B vitamins, such as riboflavin (B_1) and thiamine.

- **Biotin.** This B vitamin may improve the condition of your hair and nails.

One combination vitamin available by prescription, which I prescribe, is Encora as it contains calcium, vitamin D3 800 IU, magnesium, B vitamins, and Omega 3 all combined into two pills twice a day.

High on Exercise

You've heard of runner's high—the endorphin effect? When you exercise hard, your body releases the feel-good substances that erase the blues. By sticking to a regular exercise regimen, you'll get regular, natural boosts each week. Depending on your daytime activities—for those of us who work in cubicles, activity is probably not part of the day—you need to plan time to exercise for mental and physical health benefits.

Join a female-friendly gym if you feel uncomfortable in workout facilities; sign up for an aerobics class with a friend if you have a tendency to back out on your plans to exercise.

You don't have to run a marathon to improve your mood through exercise, however. Try a nice walk—a great way to relieve stress, enjoy a beautiful day, get some fresh air, and burn calories.

Wonder how active you really are? Wear a pedometer for a week and see how long it takes you to get in 10,000 steps a day. Taking 10,000 steps a day burns an additional 2,000–3,500 calories per week!

Lighten Up

You've probably heard of seasonal affective disorder, or SAD, a type of depression that generally sets in during winter, when days are shorter and the sky is darker. Even those of us who don't suffer from SAD can admit to feeling a bit grumpy when it rains for days in a row and sunlight is more like a golden mirage seen only on vacation.

Our bodies seem to know instinctively that exposure to bright light is important. Not only does light lift our spirits, it infuses us with the all-important vitamin D.

If natural bright light is hard to come by at home or work, think about getting your light from another source, as do some SAD patients. Light fixtures that give off 10,000 lux (a measurement of brightness) have proven effective in fighting mood disorders. These specially designed lights come in different styles—desk lamps, bedside reading lamps, even portable versions. A half hour of exposure each day increases energy and improves mood for some women. This light does *not* damage the skin or eyes like the ultraviolet rays from the sun can. Vitamin D may elevate the mood—another reason our body likes sunshine—but rather than damage the skin from too much sun exposure, I prefer for myself (and for all of my patients) to wear sunscreen and take a vitamin D3 supplement.

Caregiver Stress

Caregiver stress isn't depression, but it certainly is an emotional weight that can affect women during midlife, often coinciding with menopause.

In our society, women are socialized to be caregivers who put other people's needs first. Then, in midlife, we are often sandwiched between two generations that need us: parents, who are likely to be in their 70s to 90s, and children, who are often in the turbulent throes of adolescence. Add menopause, with its disturbed sleep and the mixed hormonal messages, to the mix, and it's no wonder we're stressed to the limit.

Here are some ways to deal with caregiver stress that will help prevent a crash.

- **Put yourself first.** I know this isn't easy. We're raised to believe that taking care of ourselves is selfish. But if you don't take time to care for your basic needs, you won't have the mental or physical strength to care for your family.

- **Eat right and exercise.** The last item on your to-do list may be to fit in a workout, but it should be first. Really! Burn off stress by getting physical.

- **Don't sideline a healthy diet.** Sugar and other indulgences are tempting when everything else in life seems to be falling apart. But the end result of comforting our stress with food is added pounds—another stress to deal with.

- **Seek help.** Women constitute 90 percent of all caregivers, so you're not alone. Talk to your doctor about caregiver support groups. Check into available home-health options for your folks. Talk to family members about ways they can help you.

For more tips on being a caregiver without neglecting yourself, see appendix 4.

Remember Janet, whose story appeared at the beginning of this chapter? I'm happy to report that after putting just a few of my suggestions into place, she's feeling much better. I'll continue to monitor her mood in case we need to take any further measures. Meanwhile, here's what she told me at our last appointment.

> *When I look into the mirror now, I see a different woman from the one who looked back at me a few months ago. I've started to exercise several times a week, and I definitely eat a healthier diet. Combined with my low-dose hormone therapy, those steps seem to be lifting me out of my funk. I've even asked my husband to take more of a role with our troublesome teenager. I have more energy to help my mom, and I no longer believe that I'm flipping out.*

Chapter 5

Menopause and Appearance

Most of the time, women don't separate how they look from how they feel. Physical appearance and emotional well-being are closely related. When you dress as if you're ready for a ball, you usually feel like a queen. When you can slide into those "skinny jeans," nothing can stop you. And when you're having a "good hair day," regardless of how superficial that sounds, you just feel better.

Menopause can be associated with a number of changes in physical appearance. Skin suddenly loses elasticity, hair thins, and many curse a "meno-potbelly."

Once menopause hits, a woman's first concerns are usually with the more disruptive symptoms, such as sleep loss, dry vagina, hot flashes, and mood swings. When she gains control over these more serious matters, she may then focus on those related to looks—skin, hair, and other body concerns.

Changes in Physical Appearance

Changes in physical appearance are sometimes the most frustrating aspect of menopause, and it's no secret why. Society conditions us to focus on the exterior, and women's magazines all claim to offer numerous means to restoring lost youth. There's a reason we see so many products on the market designed to make us look and feel our best. Our culture promotes an image of beauty that's completely unrealistic.

Veronica

Wow, I am so happy, now I don't have periods or cramps anymore. I noticed, though, that my skin is dull and very dry and most concerning is that I have started to lose clumps of hair. I expected that my skin would change somewhat, but my appearance has changed so quickly.

Can you tell which of Veronica's symptoms stem from lack of estrogen or which symptoms may be a sign of something beyond menopause? When I saw Veronica in the office, in addition to a full history and physical and hormonal assessment, I wanted to be sure that her iron levels were normal. Recent research has shown that low iron levels can accelerate hair loss. When assessing for hair loss, anything more than 150 hairs in the hair brush per day is too much, where as up to 100 per day is normal. I found that Veronica was quite low in iron. The cause of this low iron was a bleeding precancerous colon polyp that was found after undergoing full evaluation and colonoscopy only because we found her iron stores were depleted/too low. After this bleeding polyp was removed, her iron stores improved when she took Repliva 21/7 (prescription iron supplement). Her hair became thicker, and with use of local skin care products, as well as a healthy diet and exercise regimen, her skin became much brighter.

When I get dressed in the morning and style my hair, I no longer have huge clumps of hair coming out. My energy is back, and I am no longer chewing on ice cubes, which Dr. Thacker told me was a sign of low iron. I am so glad that I underwent that colonoscopy, even though I thought that my low iron state was just from having years of menstrual periods. Now that I have repleted my iron, and am on multivitamins, including biotin for my skin and hair, and possess a good skin regimen, I feel so much better.

Could Hormones Help Improve My Appearance?

When my patients discuss menopause symptoms, skin and hair are often key concerns. Many women want to know if hormones can make them look better. A typical conversation might go like this:

> *Dr. Thacker, I don't really care about my bones or heart disease just now—I just want my hair and skin to look good, and that's why I want hormones.*
> *"Well, okay," I usually respond. "It's fine to care how you look. But let's check your cholesterol and bone density while you're here."*

What you see in the mirror *does* affect how you feel emotionally. If you feel better on hormones because they improve your skin and make you feel more vibrant, I will prescribe them, as long as you understand the risks and benefits and I can monitor your reactions. My belief is that the reasons a woman wants hormone treatment are personal, and they are *her* decision. (In case you couldn't tell by now, in my mind, women's health is about personal choice.)

When our culture tells us daily that appearance is important, how can we tune the message out completely? Besides, we know from experience that we feel better when we look better.

We can control the choices we make that affect how we look and feel. Real-life solutions range from medical skin care to diet to lifestyle changes and, for some, hormone therapy. We'll talk about each of them.

Skin Care

Skin can take much more abuse when it's younger. By the time women hit menopause, it doesn't heal as fast as it used to. For instance, look at what happens with cuts. Your child's cut will heal

Feeding Your Skin

There is truth in the adage "You are what you eat." If you starve your skin of important nutrients, it will show. Stock your pantry with these skin power foods:

- **Yellow and orange foods.** Vitamin A, which is found in such foods as carrots and pumpkins, benefits skin cells.
- **Berries.** Blackberries, blueberries, strawberries, and plums are high in antioxidants (substances that inhibit reactions promoted by oxygen). The phytochemicals in these fruits can protect skin from cell-damaging free radicals.
- **Fatty acids.** Salmon, walnuts, canola oil, and flaxseed contain fatty acids—omega 3 and omega 6—which support the health of skin cell membranes. The cell membrane helps the skin retain moisture.
- **Healthy oils.** Oils keep skin lubricated. Look for those labeled "cold pressed," "expeller processed," or "extra virgin." These processes ensure that oils do not lose their nutrients during processing.
- **Whole grains, cereals, turkey, and tuna.** These foods contain selenium, which protects skin cells.
- **Green teas.** The anti-inflammatory properties of green tea protect cell membranes and are beneficial to overall skin health.
- **Water.** Water hydrates the skin and helps cells remove toxins and soak in nutrients. When we are well hydrated, we sweat efficiently, cleaning and clearing the skin.

just hours later, but you'll still be wearing a Band-Aid the next day and maybe the day after. Similarly, a skin-care regimen that's appropriate for your teenage daughter probably will not suit you.

During menopause years, women may experience the following skin symptoms.

Dryness

Most women produce less oil as they age. Lack of oils in the skin causes it to send "thirst signals" in the form of all over itching or dry patches. In severe cases, women may have chronic itching.

I recommend very practical solutions, such as using an emollient lotion like Lubriderm or substituting standard bar soap, which can irritate sensitive skin, with Aveeno Moisturizing Bar with oatmeal.

If your skin is excessively dry, you are perhaps bathing too much. Arms and legs don't need to be scrubbed daily. Concentrate on cleaning only areas like the face, feet, groin, and underarms, which do need to be washed daily.

After bathing, apply a moisturizer while your body is still damp. This traps water and protects skin from losing hydration.

• • • Fast Fact • • •

The skin is the largest organ of the body.

• • •

Tender Skin

You've never had "sensitive skin," but during menopause, you may wonder whether bathing products or laundry detergents are the source of your discomfort. This is highly possible. Skin gets thinner and becomes more delicate as we age. Perfumes or cosmetics that didn't bother you before may irritate you now.

The nipples and genital skin are especially prone to adverse reactions to soaps, lotions, and other cleansing products.

If your skin is sensitive, especially if you have eczema or burning of the nipples or vulva, try wearing only white cotton undergarments. When you wash your clothes, rinse bras and underwear twice. Don't use dryer sheets; their anti-static agents can cause irritation and itching.

Adult Breakouts

At midlife it often seems as if women who breezed through puberty without a single breakout are reaching for cover-up foundation, while those of us who suffered through acne in our younger years are sometimes free and clear from acne.

Marnie Godfrey, an aesthetician who is a medical and beauty skin care specialist at Cleveland Clinic, notices this paradox frequently in her clients. And she's seeing more midlife women dealing with stress-hormone acne today than she saw in the past. (Stress-hormone acne occurs when stress-related hormones cause excess oil production that clogs pores, which become infected— in other words, develop acne.) She attributes most of this to the additional stresses on today's women from the environment and their daily lives.

Your Ideal Skin-care Regimen

What can you do about it? Many women are confused about what they really need, which is why I recommend that you see an aesthetician like Marnie. You can also adopt a skin-care regimen like the one below, which focuses on four steps:

1. Prepare
2. Correct

3. Protect

4. Stimulate

For the care of middle-aged skin, think gentle, preventive, and protective. You want to avoid harsh soaps, moisturize, exfoliate on a regular basis to get rid of dead skin cells, and protect the skin from the sun and elements.

You don't have to purchase a shelf full of products to accomplish the four steps of proper skin care. All you need is a cleanser from your drugstore (which will tend to contain less perfume and fewer additives than a product bought at a makeup counter), a sunscreen, and a color corrector or antioxidant serum to polish and brighten skin tone while deeply exfoliating.

Prepare. Clean the skin with a product free of fragrance and additives. Medical lines such as Biomedic or Obagi are the best choice because they contain concentrations of active ingredients that you cannot purchase in the same strength over the counter.

Look for an acidic cleanser with a pH lower than 5.5. Generally, liquids are better than bars.

Protect. Sunblock is an important part of good skin care at any time of life. If you live on planet Earth, you are exposed to ultraviolet rays from the sun. Ultraviolet A (UVA) rays are present all day, year-round. They can penetrate glass, and they go straight to the underlayer of the skin. UVA rays are responsible for the long-term skin damage that comes with aging.

Ultraviolet B (UVB) rays can't pass through glass, but they can tan or burn our skin. UVB rays are more intense in the summer.

So check the ingredients in your sunblock. You want a product that protects against both types of rays.

Anthelios, an exciting product, is a moisturizing cream with an ultrapotent sunscreen—mexoryl—that blocks both UVA and

UVB rays. Women who have had skin cancer, trouble with melasma (the hormonally stimulated skin pigmentation known as the "mask of pregnancy"), or simply want the best wrinkle protection should choose Anthelios or products that contain mexoryl. (I personally like the Anthelios with SPF of 60 as it not only functions like a sunscreen but also as an illuminizer/skin brightener.)

Please note: An SPF 15 moisturizer plus an SPF 15 foundation does not equal SPF 30. The math just doesn't work that way.

Correct. You may also choose to cover blemishes with a color corrector, such as concealer or foundation.

Stimulate. If you apply lots of moisturizer but still feel dry, chances are that you need to exfoliate. Your moisturizer probably can't penetrate the skin because of an excess of dead skin cells.

Exfoliating—sloughing off dead skin cells—helps skin renew itself more quickly than it does naturally. This can improve your skin's appearance and reduce pimples and blackheads, as well as allowing your moisturizer to penetrate and do its job.

Check ingredients of drugstore brands; you're looking for products that contain alpha hydroxy and beta hydroxy acids, which remove skin cells through "fine exfoliation" and shouldn't cause flaking or redness. You don't need to go to the cosmetics counter and spend a fortune for an "exclusive" serum. There are lots of affordable options on the market today.

The best solution for exfoliation, however, is to use a medical line, available by prescription only. These contain more concentrated amounts of alpha hydroxy and beta hydroxy than over-the-counter substances can provide.

Prescription products such as RETIN-A MICRO or TAZORAC exfoliate deeply; sometimes there will be peeling. This is a sign of increased blood flow and isn't a bad thing. Some women add moisturizer to these regimens to prevent the skin from peeling.

A milder form of retinoic acid derivative like Differi. 0.3 percent, may control acne, help with exfoliation, and re. fine wrinkling and is more potent than the Differin 0.1 perce. without any increase in side effects.

Copper creams and active vitamin C applied topically may help stimulate collagen formation. Aminopeptides and substances known as "kinerases" are also used in some skin-rejuvenation products.

Many women discover that their skin can glow and feel wonderful when they care for it through a combination of diet, exercise, adequate hydration, smoke avoidance, and beauty sleep, along with an excellent skin-care regimen that includes sun protection as well as some topical rejuvenation creams.

Hair

Some women notice hair loss during menopause. Thinning hair is often related to aging. By the age of 40, many women show signs of androgenetic alopecia (AGA), a common, so-called male-pattern thinning. But, as mentioned earlier, if you're losing more than 150 strands per day, you're shedding too much hair.

Hair loss in midlife can be more severe and obvious for some women, and there are a few reasons why.

Hormonal Fluctuations

Hormonal fluctuations during menopause can trigger hair loss. If women lose too much estrogen, the hair can thin. Conversely, if a woman has too much testosterone in her system, or if dipping estrogen levels result in an increase in the relative amount of testosterone and/or increased sensitivity to the effects of testosterone at the hair-follicle level, then the amount of hair loss will exceed hair growth.

Genetics

AGA or "male-patterned" hair loss is a very common reason for genetically transmitted hair loss in men and women. In AGA, the active derivative of testosterone, dihydrotesterone (DHT), tightly binds to receptors in the scalp's hair follicles, shrinks them, and makes it impossible for healthy hair to survive. Even though we don't need hair to live, it's a symbolic and important part of most women's appearance. It can be very distressing for women if their physicians shrug off their hair loss.

During menopause, as estrogen levels decline, the level of testosterone can become a powerful factor. The more testosterone, the more DHT and the more possible hair loss. Pre-existing AGA can get worse at the time of menopause or any hormonal perturbation.

Women with AGA do not become entirely bald, as men with AGA do. That being said, the condition is still challenging.

Medical Side Effects

Another reason for hair loss may be the use of certain medications. These include medications used to treat high blood pressure, heart problems, depression, or gout; the chemotherapy or radiation treatments given to cancer patients; and in some cases, unusually high levels of vitamin A or low levels of iron or protein.

Illness

Finally, hair loss can be caused by unrelated illnesses, including thyroid disease, severe infection or flu, or fungal infections such as ringworm of the scalp, all of which have nothing to do with menopause.

What Can I Do If I'm Experiencing Hair Loss?

First of all, you need to find a physician who is interested in hair loss. This might be a dermatologist or a hormone specialist. You need a thorough evaluation of your skin, hair, nutrition, hormones, and medical circumstances.

Most women benefit from vitamins such as Biotin Forte and iron, as well as a healthy diet and balanced hormonal status. Shampoos such as Nizoral can block DHT production in the hair follicle. Rogaine HP (an over-the-counter medication that you apply to hair) can treat androgenetic alopecia, but you must use it faithfully for six months before you'll know if it will help restore your hair growth, and it can be messy and inconvenient.

I tend to favor oral estrogen therapy for menopausal women concerned about skin and hair changes because this increases the liver's production of sex hormone-binding globulin (SHBG), and when SHBG levels rise, there is less active, free testosterone to diffuse into skin structures.

Spironolactone, a potassium-sparing diuretic, blocks the effects of DHT on the hair follicle and produces improvements in both acne and hair-thinning. However, in pre- or perimenopausal women, spironolactone has been associated with menstrual disturbance, so many times either hormonal contraception or hormonal therapy is used in conjunction with spironolactone.

Several years ago, a novel form of a progestogen, drospirenone (DRSP), was developed. Under the name of YASMIN, it quickly became the most popular birth control pill worldwide because its DRSP causes neither weight gain nor bloating and because as a spironolactone analogue, it has favorable effects on the skin and hair. In 2006, YAZ, a lower-dose version of YASMIN, became available for both hormonal contraception and acne treatment in women, and has become a very popular hormonal agent. YAZ is also the first hormone pill that the FDA has approved for the treatment of severe PMS.

Rather than prescribe a hormonal contraceptive (HC) agent and spironolactone, I frequently select YASMIN or YAZ for women who are concerned about their skin and hair.

Most recently, women were given a new postmenopausal HT regimen option that contains estradiol and DRSP in pill form, called ANGELIQ.

If you have exhausted all the medical, nutritional, hormonal, and dermatological treatments for hair loss, then in severe cases you may wish to explore hair replacement procedures such as grafting. A dermatological surgeon can determine whether your case is appropriate for such treatment and can perform these outpatient procedures, but you must undergo medical evaluation first.

I have one clever and stylish patient who discovered that with creative hairstyling and tinted hairspray to match her hair color, no telltale scalp could be seen.

Weight

It's a fact of life: Your metabolism will slow down as you get older. Declining hormones eat away muscle mass, and muscle burns more calories than fat mass. No wonder women tend to gain 10 to 15 pounds at midlife. The harsh reality is that at this age, burning calories and keeping off extra weight simply takes more work.

If a pill could reverse metabolic slowdown or make our bodies burn calories while we relax on the couch, most Americans would pay handsomely for it.

The bad news? There's no such thing. The only way to combat weight gain is to reduce caloric intake and boost exercise.

We'll talk more about nutrition, vitamins, and healthy eating for life in chapter 6. For now, we'll focus on getting physical and why no woman can ignore the importance of regular exercise.

Work Out a Plan

Exercise doesn't have to mean marathon training or bulking up at the gym. Sure, the goal is to build lean muscle mass, and the way to do this is by lifting weights. And you need to burn calories, which is accomplished by running, walking, and many other aerobic activities.

But you want to set realistic fitness goals, so think first about what you enjoy. After all, you'll want to stick with your program, and if you can't stand the thought of running laps on a track, you won't last more than a week.

Read and Get Inspired

There are shelves of books on the subject of exercise. Depending on your interests, you may reach for a yoga guide or a weight-loss success story. The point is to inspire yourself to be good to your body.

I recommend both *Body for Life for Women: A Woman's Plan for Physical and Mental Transformation* by Dr. Pamela Peeke and *Weigh Less, Live Longer: Dr. Lou Aronne's "Getting Healthy" Plan for Permanent Weight Control* by Dr. Louis J. Aronne.

Every woman's fitness goals are different, so explore the library for books that speak to your exercise and weight-loss needs.

But don't just read about it. It's all too easy for some of us to do the research and keep putting off the footwork. Remember, you need to *do* it.

Group Work

For many women, having an exercise buddy or hearing encouragement from a friend is what gets them to a workout. If this describes you, consider signing up for exercise classes with a friend.

Try Pilates, which is a great form of stretching and strengthening exercise. Venture into kickboxing, tai chi, water aerobics—any activity that sounds interesting and will hold your attention.

Variety in workouts also tones different muscle groups and prevents boredom. And by signing up with a friend or family member, you are less likely to come up with excuses to skip class.

Women-friendly Gyms

Many women feel more comfortable in a same-sex environment. If this is you, consider joining a gym like Curves.

Take the Long Route

If you want to incorporate exercise into your lifestyle, think of little things you can do to increase your cardio levels throughout the day. Take the stairs. Park your car far away from building entrances and walk across the lots. Power walk for ten minutes before work, during lunch, and in the evening—that's thirty minutes total. Research has shown that even little spurts of activity count.

Track Your Steps

Consider buying a pedometer and make sure you walk 10,000 steps each day. (Several recent research studies have concluded that walking this distance daily provides substantial health benefits.)

You might be surprised to find, as I did, that on days you feel extremely tired, you've walked the least. When I started tracking my steps, I discovered that if I was seeing patients in my office all day, I might feel exhausted by the time I drove home. Mentally, I had run miles. But actually, my physical activity was way below the 10,000-step goal I had set.

On the other hand, when I'm literally running errands, exercising during my sons' sports practices, or grocery shopping and taking care of chores around the house, I'll rack up 10,000 steps easily because I'm not sitting. It pays to keep track and increase your activity as necessary. On days you think you'll fall short, fit an extra walk in during lunch, plan to go to the gym in the evening, walk nine holes of golf, or make a tennis date! When I'm wearing my pedometer, I am more motivated to take the stairs and walk the extra distance at work because I know I have a target to reach.

Learn to Relax

Many physical disorders are stress related, including ulcers, headaches, and back pain. In addition, when we're stressed, our bodies produce the hormone cortisol. There's a link between high levels of cortisol and abdominal fat, which is the worst kind of fat to have because it increases your risk of heart disease and stroke far more than when body fat is below the belly.

What's more, stress is a sneaky stumbling block in our plans to exercise and eat well. "I don't have time to prepare a healthy meal," and "I can't squeeze a workout into my schedule today," might sound familiar to you.

Relaxation isn't a natural activity for many of us. We're programmed to go, go, go. But we must learn how to wind down, breathe deeply, and block out distracting thoughts. When we make time to do this, we're feeding our bodies with the quiet time they need.

Just think of all the ordinary stresses you encounter every day. Then add in the stresses of menopause and midlife, and you'll quickly realize why relaxation is such an important part of a healthful daily routine.

Try the relaxation techniques listed here. See which ones you enjoy the most. Then plan time to relax at least once a day, even if it's just for a few minutes. Twice a day, morning and evening, would be even better, if your schedule allows. (But please, don't get stressed out about having enough time to relax!)

Relaxation Techniques. Here are a few relaxation exercises you can try (adapted from "Relaxation and Other Alternative Approaches for Managing Headaches," Cleveland Clinic Health Information Center, *http://my.clevelandclinic.org/disorders/Headaches/*). I find that when patients with severe menopause symptoms practice relaxation techniques, they feel that they have more control over their bodies and lives.

Rhythmic breathing. If your breathing is short and hurried, slow it down by taking long, slow breaths. Inhale slowly. Then exhale slowly, paying attention to the way your body naturally relaxes. Recognizing this change will help you relax more. I recommend taking several deep, cleansing breaths. I do this at least once every time I look at my watch and realize that I'm running late.

Deep breathing. Imagine a spot just below your navel. Breathe into that spot, filling your abdomen with air, then let it out slowly. Each time you exhale, you should feel more relaxed.

Visualized breathing. Combine slow breathing with your imagination. Picture relaxation entering your body and tension leaving your body. Breathe deeply but naturally.

As you inhale, visualize air entering your nostrils, traveling to your lungs, and expanding your chest and abdomen. As you exhale, visualize your breath leaving your body. Every time you inhale, imagine that you're breathing in more relaxation. Every time you exhale, see yourself breathing out stress.

Progressive muscle relaxation. After taking a few deep breaths, mentally scan your body for areas that are tense and cramped. Loosen each area by tensing it and then releasing the tension.

Rotate your head in a smooth motion once or twice. Roll your shoulders forward and backward several times. Let all your muscles completely relax. Recall a pleasant thought for a few seconds, take a few more deep breaths, and exhale.

Relax to music. Combine any of these relaxation exercises with your favorite relaxing or mood-lifting music playing softly in the background.

Mental imagery. Guided imagery helps create harmony between the mind and body. Think of it as a "mental escape." There are many guided imagery CDs and cassettes for sale.

Positive self-talk. Identify negative self-talk and concentrate on positive, healthy self-talk. Use affirmations to counteract negative thoughts and emotions. Try repeating positive statements, such as "I am healthy, vital, and strong," "There is nothing in the world I cannot handle," "I let go of things I cannot control," and "Every day I'm getting stronger."

It's Your Choice

In many respects, your health and how you feel about yourself are your choice. Certainly, the decisions you make concerning your appearance, weight, fitness, and ability to relax affect how you look and feel not only now but later in life.

Some women just don't seem to get this connection. I see women who eat only organic foods but smoke; workout nuts who reward themselves with desserts that contain twice the calories they burn; menopausal women, terrified by the exaggerated risks of hormone therapy, who gobble tons of herbs, supplements, and other unregu-lated concoctions that have never been rigorously tested, monitored, or studied; women afraid to undergo proven screening tests who don't take the time to buckle their seatbelts when they get into the car.

Don't fall prey to such misguided thinking. Follow the advice in this book and refer to it often. Stick with proven techniques to help yourself look and feel your best and don't ignore warnings about the less-than-safe health practices some women adopt.

Changes to skin, weight, and other physical attributes may occur gradually, or they may seem to appear out of nowhere. Caring for yourself and dealing with these changes in a positive fashion give you an opportunity to make your health and happiness a priority.

Take care of your skin and hair. Use whatever remedies work well for you. But don't let our culture's perverse obsession with youthful appearance force you to feel bad about the fact that you're maturing.

Choose an approach to exercise that fits your lifestyle. Be sure to add some weight-bearing, muscle-building activities. And don't forget to relax deeply and often. It's good for you and those around you.

Talk to your doctor about hormone therapy and find out whether you need it. You have your whole life left to live. You might as well look and feel good living it.

Chapter 6

Healthy Nutrition for a Healthy Midlife

Nutrition is vitally important at midlife. Why? Well, our metabolism is slowing, our muscle mass is decreasing, and we can't rebound from the consequences of poor health choices, like eating fast food or drinking too much, the way we might have in our 20s and 30s.

More important, what we eat affects many of the body organs and physical processes that are further affected by our declining levels of estrogen. Our choice of foods, vitamins, and supplements impacts the heart, brain, and bones and influence disease prevention—even hot flashes in some cases.

I like to think of midlife as a sort of reset button. These years are your chance to play with destiny and really control how you will look and feel for the next forty years or more by making those wise nutritional choices, one bite at a time.

My patient Louise learned firsthand how life changing a move toward good nutrition can be.

Louise

When I entered menopause early after I had a hysterectomy at age 39, my body seemed to soak up fat and calories because of my slower metabolism, lack of exercise, and just plain old overeating. I was already very overweight, so this was daunting.

Lack of estrogen after my ovaries were removed seemed to cause my already elevated weight to surge. In addition, I had severe hot flashes, and my bones seemed very fragile; I even broke an arm. Without any estrogen, my body seemed to have a mind of its own, and it kept playing tricks on me.

I searched the website of the North American Menopause Society for a specialist in menopause and found Dr. Thacker, who prescribed hormone therapy. It really helped. But it was hard to actually feel good about myself when I was so overweight.

I deserved better. I owed it to myself to lose the weight. It was a good time to seriously reconsider my lifestyle, and this time, I had a free pass from my insurance company to take care of business. At 100 pounds over my ideal body weight, I was approved for bariatric surgery. The procedure would have shaved off more than a third of the old Louise.

But all my life, taking shortcuts has never paid off. I decided not to have the bariatric surgery. Instead, I started seeing a nutritionist, as Dr. Thacker recommended, for advice about my diet.

I learned everything I needed to know about nutrition at midlife. My nutritionist explained good and bad food choices, introduced me to the Food Guide Pyramid, advised me about portion control, informed me about foods said to help menopausal women, and explained the role of regular exercise.

As I tackled the pretty radical changes in my diet, I focused on the fact that the choice was mine. As Dr. Thacker told me, a healthy lifestyle is a choice.

I was eating fewer calories—mainly whole grains, fruits, and vegetables—and choosing lean proteins like fish. The weight began to come off. Every pound I lost was an added incentive to lose more.

At the beginning, Dr. Thacker prescribed XENICAL (orlistat), the fat blocker, to help me. If I cheated on my diet and ate too much, I had to run for the bathroom and, once there . . . well, I'll spare you the details. Suffice it to say, I didn't cheat often. I also exercised daily for an hour.

After I was off the medication, when I found myself wanting Kentucky Fried Chicken for dinner or a big bowl of ice cream for a snack, I reminded myself that I was doing this for me.

I'm 100 pounds lighter now and so happy. I feel as if I've shed my old self, and I really like how I look and feel.

Note: I don't usually prescribe XENICAL, a fat blocker, unless my patient is overweight. It's relatively expensive, and it's FDA approved only for people with a body mass index of 27 or more. When I do prescribe it, it is a temporary measure. I use it only as tool to boost the weight loss plan of someone who's really working hard at reducing calories and exercising regularly. The product ALLI is the same substance as XENICAL and is now available without a prescription.

Two years after deciding against bariatric surgery, Louise came for an appointment looking absolutely fabulous. Her entire disposition was different. She was lighthearted, confident, and clearly loving life. I tell Louise's story as often as I can to inspire others.

She came to see me to get a clean bill of health because she had found a new partner. Her new appearance had boosted her self-esteem and given her a certain poise that she lacked when she carried all that extra weight. And the result was that after being alone for what she described as "way too long," she had found romance.

Louise changed her habits dramatically. We all have to do that if we want to stay healthy and vibrant throughout our midlife years and beyond.

Climbing the Pyramid

The mission of the Center for Nutrition Policy and Promotion, an agency of the U.S. Department of Agriculture, is to improve the nutrition and well-being of Americans. The most recent version of the Food Guide Pyramid, a guide to food choices, can be found at *www.mypyramid.gov.*

The site offers a multicolored pyramid, each level of which represents a particular food group. There are also useful tips to help you rearrange your eating habits for a healthier you. Some examples include these:

- Make half your grains whole.
- Vary your veggies.
- Focus on fruit.
- Get your calcium-rich foods.
- Go lean with protein.
- Find your balance between food and physical activity.

Weight-attracting Danger Zones

Women are most likely to gain weight at certain times that often coincide with the midlife years. These "danger zones" include the following:

- Times when women are sleep-deprived (such as from disruptive hot flashes and night sweats).

Can Not Sleeping Make You Fat?

Studies show that people who don't sleep enough are more prone to weight gain than those who get plenty of shut-eye. The reason is that the hormone levels regulating appetite are governed in part by sleep. When you don't get enough rest, there aren't enough hormones present telling you that you just ate. So you keep eating. And so the weight goes on, and on, and on.

If you're trying to lose or maintain weight, be sure to get enough sleep.

- Times when stress hormones are on high alert.

- Periods of life change, good or bad, including weddings, birth, death, divorce, an empty nest, and when experiencing issues with aging parents.

An overload of stress can eat away at willpower to avoid "bad" foods.

What Is the Ideal Weight-loss Diet?

The diet industry is rich with ways for us to zap fat, lose weight before the weekend, stay slim forever, and drop pounds without lifting a finger. Yeah, right.

The fact is, to lose weight, the old input-output equation still holds true. You must burn more calories than you consume. You can't trick your body by trying any other approach. It will know! And even if you lose weight, it will come right back when you return to your usual eating habits.

Eating programs work differently for everyone. One person may thrive on a high-protein diet; another may function best with more carbohydrates. It's not easy to tell ahead of time which diet will work for you.

When pressed to recommend a plan that works, I endorse the Mediterranean diet. This way of eating includes lots of fruits and vegetables, with some whole grain bread and other cereals, potatoes, beans, nuts, and seeds. Olive oil is the fat used most often. The diet also includes dairy products, fish, and poultry in small to moderate amounts, with very little red meat.

Studies of people who follow the Mediterranean diet show that they tend to be healthier, live longer, and have less chronic disease than typical Americans.

The bottom-line: Adopt a heart-healthy diet, high in vegetables and whole grains and free of all trans fats.

What's the Difference Between Saturated Fats and Trans Fats?

Both are key dietary factors in elevating cholesterol, but they're found in different foods.

Saturated fats are usually solid at room temperature—they don't combine well with oxygen. They raise your total cholesterol level as well as your LDL ("bad") cholesterol. You'll find saturated fats in foods that come from animals, such as whole milk, cream, butter, cheese, lard, and meats.

Trans fats are usually created through partial hydrogenation, a process that heats vegetable oil and transforms it under pressure. This makes the oils easier to use in food production and gives processed food a longer shelf life. These fats are found in many commercially packaged foods, such as potato chips, cookies, crackers, microwave popcorn, cakes, French fries, and doughnuts.

Trans fats pack a double whammy. They can raise bad cholesterol and lower good cholesterol. They are so unhealthy that the American Heart Association's Nutrition Committee strongly

The "Low-fat" Phenomenon

"Low-fat" on the label doesn't translate to "healthy." Cotton candy contains no fat, but it's not good for you. Cookies, cakes, and snack foods that advertise as "low-fat" are just that. But they aren't low in calories, and they're certainly not a replacement for healthful snacks, such as fruits, nuts, or veggies.

Some women wonder why they don't shed pounds on low-fat diets, and I tell them to examine their food choices. You can have a horrible diet that is low-fat. Or your low-carb diet may be polluted with trans fats. Healthy eating is about balance and choosing the right foods.

Cutting back fat without also cutting calories will get you nowhere.

advises limiting the intake of trans fat to less than 1 percent of total calories daily.

Food for Thought

There are lots of misconceptions out there about foods that heal, and my patients ask me about nutrition all the time.

It seems that no one can resist sounding off on what we should eat and why. We hear from the media, medical community, dietitians, and even celebrities and self-proclaimed specialists whose research may be no deeper than the Web page where they spout their nutritional advice. We hear mixed messages about soy, organic foods, and supplements. What are we supposed to believe? It's hard to know whom to trust.

The questions below crop up daily in my discussions with women. Here are my thoughts on these crucial topics.

Will Hormone Therapy Make Me Fat?

No! Low-dose hormone therapy does not cause weight gain. Several randomized trials have shown that women who take placebos gain more weight than women on estrogen. I find that many of my patients actually lose a slight amount of weight when they start taking estrogen because they feel better and sleep better.

Our metabolic rate slows as we age, so women who do not compensate for this by reducing calories and exercising will gain weight. Hormone therapy isn't the culprit. Poor diet and lack of exercise are.

Is There a Menopause Diet?

This is a disputed topic. Many so-called health experts claim that you can alleviate menopause symptoms with certain foods or supplements. But some risk factors associated with aging and menopause can't be changed. Nonetheless, healthy eating can help prevent or reduce the bothersome symptoms that women develop during and after menopause. (See my recommendations on page 110.)

Will Soy Products Relieve Menopause Symptoms?

Soy is a rich source of phytoestrogens, plant-derived compounds that can behave like estrogen in the body. In some women, soy metabolizes into equol, a weak estrogen.

But there's a catch. Not every woman's body converts soy into equol, so not all of us would benefit from including more soy in our diets.

Then why all the buzz about soy? There are two main reasons.

Studies show that Asian women who eat a lot of soy tend to have fewer hot flashes and lower rates of breast cancer than

American women. And research performed on primates has produced results indicating that soy may have some cardiovascular benefits.

But there are snags with both claims.

Snag #1: Soy does not dissipate all menopausal side effects, even in Asian women. Despite reduced hot flashes, these women still experience vaginal dryness and are at risk for bone thinning and eventual bone loss.

Snag #2: Monkeys convert soy food into equol more efficiently than human beings do, so primate-based research does not translate into the same outcome for all women.

Soy foods may have some health benefits, but they may not apply to all people. Don't fill your pantry with soy powders, shakes, bars, and especially soy pills in the hope of alleviating all menopause symptoms. Even if your body converts soy into equol, you may not be addressing every menopause-related health problem. Furthermore, soy pills may or may not contain high doses of isoflavones, a class of phytoestrogens, and they do not contain the soy protein part of the food. For these reasons, they are not recommended as menopause therapy.

Of course, go ahead and eat soy foods if you like the taste of them. But stay away from the other soy-related items out there.

Will Eating Soy Affect My Cholesterol Levels?

Research shows that 25 grams of soy food per day may reduce cholesterol levels. Women who prefer natural remedies to prescription medication for lowering mild elevations in cholesterol may incorporate soy foods into their diets, along with oat bran, apple pectins, and garlic, and see improved cholesterol results. Reducing trans fats and reducing any extra body weight will also help in improving cholesterol levels.

Can Women Who Have Had Breast Cancer Eat Soy?

If you are a breast cancer survivor and you like soy milk, nuts, and other whole-food products that contain soy, enjoy them in moderation. Do not take soy supplements.

I do not recommend that *any* woman take soy supplement pills—it's the whole food that is healthy, not some high-dose extraction of a part of the food.

Do I Need to Buy Cereals, Bars, and Drinks Labeled "For Women?"

If they taste good, go ahead and buy them. But keep in mind that labels are marketing tools, and most cereals and bars that are "good for women" are healthy for everyone. Many of them contain calcium, antioxidants, B vitamins, or folic acid.

A better way to go would be to find foods you like that naturally contain these nutrients. For example, broccoli is high in calcium and has cancer-fighting properties. (Go to *www.mypyramid.gov* for a list of nutrient-rich foods.)

What Is Flaxseed, and Why Do I Need It?

Flaxseed contains omega-3 essential fat, the same kind of beneficial fat found in salmon and tuna as well as almonds and walnuts. I recommend eating fish at least once or twice a week for the omega-3s, but if you don't like fish, be sure to try flaxseed.

Flaxseed contains lignans, which are believed to be anticancer agents. Flaxseed, like soy foods, may not affect menopausal symptoms, but it may help lower cholesterol.

I like ground flaxseed, flax bread, and cereal rather than flaxseed oil because whole foods are also a great source of fiber. You can grind flax seeds in a coffee grinder. Some women like to mix a small scoop into yogurt or smoothies.

Should I Avoid Certain Foods While I Am Going Through Menopause?

If you experience hot flashes, avoid spicy foods, hot beverages, caffeine, and alcohol, which can aggravate symptoms in some women. On the other hand, spices add lots of flavor without adding extra calories. So test yourself. If you flash after eating a hot tamale taco, cool it with the extra spice.

Can I Eat Red Meat?

It's a good idea to reduce the amount of red meat you eat to maintain healthy cholesterol levels and lower your risk of heart disease. Some studies show that women with daily consumption of red meat have more uterine fibroids. And because some livestock are fed hormones to promote growth, you may consume secondhand hormones in your steak dinner. Taken in small amounts, this generally will not affect most women, but why expose yourself to any unnecessary risk?

Some lean red meat is healthy for women because it contains iron, protein, and zinc. Moderation is the key. If your cholesterol is normal, then eating red meat once or twice a week is fine. However, one can maintain very good nutrition without any meat intake at all. A good nutritionist can guide you to a balanced, healthy diet designed for you individually. The focus should be on getting lots of fruits and vegetables, since they contain a number of phytonutrients that fight cancer.

The key is to eat a wide variety of fruits and vegetables, whether organic or conventional, and always wash produce thoroughly.

Menu "Musts" for Midlife

A colorful plate is the sign of a nutritious meal. If you fill your plate with food that is green, red (antioxidants), brown (grains), and white (dairy), you're on your way to fulfilling the government's My Pyramid guidelines.

But midlife women have some extra needs not covered in the guidelines. We need an extra boost in the calcium and iron departments. Meanwhile, avoiding trans fats becomes even more important to us once we're monitoring our cholesterol and taking preventive measures to reduce the risk of cancer and other diseases. And because our metabolic rate slows, portion control has never been so critical.

Here are some extra diet guidelines for midlife women. Copy this section and post it on your refrigerator or bring it with you to the grocery store.

When healthy eating becomes a habit, it won't seem like a chore.

Whole Grains, Fruits, and Veggies

Make this triad your mainstay. (Women with gluten intolerance/celiac disease must avoid all wheat and gluten protein. Fortunately, they have a number of good alternatives, so even if you're sensitive to gluten there are still some breads and pastas you can enjoy.)

"Good" Oils and Fats

Favor olive oil or canola oil over vegetable oils. Avoid saturated and trans fats, and choose foods with omega-3s, such as salmon, almonds, and flaxseed.

Soy Foods

Even though soy pills are not a menopause "solution," soy foods are still healthful. Always choose whole soy foods and not soy pills or powders. Try tofu, soy nuts, soy milk, or soy burgers. Soy pills and powders *are not to be used.* They have been associated with endometrial hyperplasia (tissue overgrowth that can be a precursor to uterine cancer).

Calcium

Eat or drink three to four servings of dairy products and calcium-rich foods a day. Find calcium in dairy, fish with bones (sardines and canned salmon), broccoli, and legumes like peas or beans.

But don't rely on foods to fulfill your daily calcium requirement. Most women simply do not get enough calcium from their diet. Others are lactose intolerant and avoid dairy products. As discussed in chapter 3, unless you drink a quart of skim milk daily (and I'm guessing you don't), take a calcium supplement to reach the recommended daily amount of 1,200 mg. (Most women only ingest 600 mg daily—half the amount they need.) Women older than age 55 who are not on estrogen absorb less calcium from their diet, so they need to ingest 1,500 mg of calcium daily.

Where to Find Calcium. The chart below features some calcium-rich foods.

FOOD, STANDARD SERVING	CALCIUM (in milligrams, mg)
DAIRY SOURCES	
Yogurt	
Plain, nonfat, 8 oz	452
Plain, low-fat, 8 oz	415
Fruit, low-fat, 8 oz	345
Plain, whole milk, 8 oz	285

Cheese

Romano cheese, 1.5 oz	452
Muenster cheese, 1.5 oz	415
Swiss cheese, 1.5 oz	336
Provolone cheese, 1.5 oz	321
Mozzarella cheese, part-skim, 1.5 oz	311
Cheddar cheese, 1.5 oz	307
Blue cheese, 1.5 oz	225
Feta cheese, 1.5 oz	210

Milk

Skim milk, 1 cup	300
1 percent low-fat milk, 1 cup	290
1 percent low-fat chocolate milk, 1 cup	288
2 percent reduced-fat milk, 1 cup	285
2 percent reduced-fat chocolate milk, 1 cup	285
Buttermilk, low-fat, 1 cup	284
Chocolate milk, 1 cup	280
Whole milk, 1 cup	276

NONDAIRY SOURCES

Seaweed, agar, dried, 3.5 oz	625
Tofu, calcium-fortified, ½ cup	424
Canned salmon, with edible bones, 3 oz	324
Sesame seeds, dried and roasted, 1 tablespoon	281
Calcium-fortified orange juice, 6 oz	200
Black-eyed peas, boiled, 1 cup	161
Spinach, cooked, ½ cup	120
Raisins, ⅔ cup	49
Butternut squash, boiled, ½ cup	42
Broccoli, boiled, ½ cup	36

Calcium With Convenience

Calcium supplements come in two forms: calcium carbonate and calcium citrate. Calcium citrate is acid-based and calcium carbonate is alkaline-based. Both types are effective.

I recommend calcium citrate. One reason is simple convenience. You can take it with or without food, whereas calcium carbonate should be taken with food to improve absorption. Also, calcium citrate absorbs into your system better than calcium carbonate does, and it has not been associated with a higher risk of kidney stones.

However, calcium citrate costs more than calcium carbonate, so if budget is an issue, feel free to take calcium carbonate and know that it works well.

Vitamin D

Calcium builds strong bones, but it isn't absorbed well without vitamin D. All women need to get enough vitamin D; in northern climates with less sun exposure, this can be especially hard to do. If you follow the reference daily intake (RDI) and take only 400 IU, you're only getting enough vitamin D to prevent rickets. (RDI is the new term for RDA, recommended dietary allowance.) Most bone experts recommend 800 to 1,000 IU of vitamin D daily. People who have been low in vitamin D need at least 2,000 IU of vitamin D3 daily.

Getting enough vitamin D has been associated with reduced risks for breast, colon, pancreas, and prostate cancer, as well as diabetes, arthritis, osteoporosis, multiple sclerosis, and falls. Far too many people are deficient in vitamin D. Your vitamin D level should be over 31 and closer to 50. Results for most of the women I test are well below these levels.

Be sure to pay attention to calcium *and* vitamin D daily.

Iron and Vitamin C

Women lose 15 to 20 mg of iron each month during menstruation. Even if you are past having periods, iron is still vital. The RDI is 18 mg up to age 50 and 10 mg after that.

Too much iron can cause problems with iron overload, and a small percentage of people absorb too much iron and have hemochromatosis (a buildup of iron in the liver that can lead to liver enlargement). Once menstruation ceases, the extra iron in "women's formulation" vitamins is usually no longer needed.

Most women absorb only 15 percent of the iron in their regular diet. If you eat some vitamin C with iron-bearing food, the amount you absorb will increase.

Iron is abundant in such foods as lean red meat, potatoes, leafy green vegetables, iron-fortified cereals, and blackstrap molasses.

Where to Find Iron. The chart below features more iron-rich foods. It's Available at *www.health.gov/dietaryguidelines/dga2005/ document/html/appendixB.htm.*

FOOD, STANDARD SERVING	IRON (in milligrams, mg)
Clams, canned, drained, 3 oz	23.8
Fortified ready-to-eat cereals (various)	1.8–21.1
1 oz Oysters, eastern, wild, cooked, 3 oz	10.2
Organ meats (liver, giblets), various, cooked, 3 oz *	5.2–9.9
Fortified instant cooked cereals (various), 1 packet	4.9–8.1
Soybeans, mature, cooked, ½ cup	4.4
Pumpkin and squash seed kernels, roasted, 1 oz	4.2
White beans, canned, ½ cup	3.9

Blackstrap molasses, 1 tbsp	3.5
Lentils, cooked, ½ cup	3.3
Spinach, fresh, cooked, ½ cup	3.2
Beef, chuck, blade roast, lean, cooked, 3 oz	3.1
Beef, bottom round, lean, 0" fat, all grades, cooked, 3 oz	2.8
Kidney beans, cooked, ½ cup	2.6
Sardines, canned in oil, drained, 3 oz	2.5
Beef, rib, lean, ¼" fat, all grades, 3 oz	2.4
Chickpeas, cooked, ½ cup	2.4
Duck, meat only, roasted, 3 oz	2.3
Lamb, shoulder, arm, lean, ¼" fat, choice, cooked, 3 oz	2.3
Prune juice, ¾ cup	2.3
Shrimp, canned, 3 oz	2.3
Cowpeas, cooked, ½ cup	2.2
Ground beef, 15 percent fat, cooked, 3 oz	2.2
Tomato purée, ½ cup	2.2
Lima beans, cooked, ½ cup	2.2
Soybeans, green, cooked, ½ cup	2.2
Navy beans, cooked, ½ cup	2.1
Refried beans, ½ cup	2.1
Beef, top sirloin, lean, 0" fat, all grades, cooked, 3 oz	2.0
Tomato paste, ¼ cup	2.0

* High in cholesterol

• • • *Fast Fact* • • •

Shopping at the periphery of your grocery store
can help improve your diet. That's where you'll find
produce, low-fat meats, and dairy items while
avoiding the junk foods and processed foods sold
in the middle of the market.

• • •

Should You Supplement?

Popping a pill that includes the nutrients of every woman-friendly food is far more convenient (and maybe more appealing) than filling up on spinach, salmon, antioxidant-rich berries, and other power foods. Many women want extracts and oils rather than real food. They figure, "Why eat your carrots if you can take a beta-carotene supplement?"

The answer is simple. Nature intended us to consume nutrients in the form of whole foods. Eating whole foods gives the body the best chance to absorb the right nutrients and process them effectively for the strongest health benefits. Whole foods come first, with supplements providing more of the vitamins and minerals that women may need.

While is it advisable and beneficial for most women to take some supplements to reach necessary levels of calcium and especially vitamin D, the supplements are a support, not a complete solution in a bottle.

Remember that in general, even high-quality supplements cannot replace the health benefits of eating nutritious food.

What If I Don't Have Time to Prepare a Healthy Meal?

If you feel that finding the time to shop for and prepare a healthy meal is impossible, you're not alone. Many of us have hectic

The Indulgence Diet (for Chocolate Lovers)

You can enjoy chocolate and even alcohol in moderation. You've probably read this in magazines, but this time the claim is 100 percent medically accurate—at least, it's accurate if you're talking about dark chocolate and red wine.

Dark chocolate is rich in arginine, a heart-smart amino acid, and for some people it has mild mood-elevating properties. Red wine is loaded with flavonoids, which have antioxidant properties.

But don't overdo either of them. Too much chocolate may go to your waistline. And too much wine will still make you drunk (and in the long term will damage your liver, heart, and brain).

schedules and feel as if we can't find time to get to the grocery store, let alone pick out appropriate foods and then cook a nutritious dinner. With alarming frequency, drive-through meals have become common fare, and the family dinner has become a rarity.

We have to change the way we think about mealtime. Eating really is a matter of life or death, and this means consuming nutritious foods, not dining at the first fast-food place you see on the way home.

I'm sure that with a little shuffling of priorities, you can schedule a time to shop for groceries and set aside a couple of hours on the weekend to prepare for the coming week.

Here are some healthful ideas:

- Cut lots of vegetables ahead of time for salads, side dishes, and quick snacks. Store them in plastic bags.

- Prepare a meal you can reinvent the next night. (Stir-fry makes a nice filling for a next-day omelet; a casserole freezes well for later in the week.)

- Store a couple of healthy frozen dinners in your freezer for lunches or dinners.

- Pack meal supplements like nutrition bars for lunches on the run.

- If you don't have time to eat breakfast, drink it in the form of Boost, Ensure, or other meal-replacement beverages.

- Purchase portion-controlled snack packs so you can munch between meals without consuming too many calories. There are several brands that make "100-calorie packs."

- Bananas are great on-the-go snacks. So are apples, nuts, and dried fruits.

- Take turns planning meals. If every person in your household is responsible for dinner once or twice a week, the whole family learns how to plan and prepare healthy meals.

The key is not to let yourself get too hungry and to be honest about your lifestyle. When you know you won't have time to prepare a nutritious meal, go ahead and take a shortcut. Just make it a healthy one.

Chapter 7

Hot Flashes and Night Sweats

I f there's one line that screams menopause (inevitably a hot topic in personal conversations among midlife women), it's *I'm having a hot flash!*

There's no mistaking the sudden intense wave of heat, rapid heartbeat, and—depending on the severity—dizziness, sweating, nausea, and feeling of weakness. Surely, you're going to suffocate. Someone open a window!

You flap your arms wildly in an attempt to fan away the perspiration that collects first on your upper lip, then your forehead and neck. Sometimes it's an all-out soaker. This is never good, especially if the episode occurs during a board meeting or leaves you with soggy sheets in the middle of the night.

Hot flashes are even more upsetting if they happen up to thirty or more times a day, as they did with Linda. I have known Linda for more than ten years, and before she began taking estrogen therapy, her hot flashes greatly interfered with everyday life. Just listen to her description.

Linda

I am the chief financial officer of my company, and my episodes are downright embarrassing—and horribly frequent. I can't get through a one-hour meeting without arousing the concern of others at the table.

I turn tomato red. My temperature rises what seems like 30 degrees—I could swear I'm in the Sahara. This lasts for up to five minutes. Then I break into a sweat and my face loses all color. This happens up to thirty or more times a day!

It's highly disruptive at work, and it's just as disturbing at night when I'm trying to sleep. I just can't get a good night's rest. Every time I have another flash, I wake up, my heart pounding. Sometimes I feel as if someone is smothering me with an electric blanket cranked up to the highest setting. I can soak the bed with perspiration. After particularly bad episodes, I have to change my nightgown and my sheets.

Linda's case is extreme, but most women experience hot flashes to some extent during the years of menopause. Often occurring at night, the hot flashes are uncomfortable and almost always accompanied by perspiration, the body's natural coolant.

I prescribed hormone therapy for Linda, and her frequent, soaking flashes were history.

What Exactly Is a Hot Flash?

A hot flash is a discrete episode of intense heat that starts at the chest and neck, flows to the head, and lasts several minutes. *Flash* is the key word. It happens suddenly and lasts only minutes. A flash is accompanied by perspiration and is an entirely different sensation from just "feeling hot."

Some women who complain of hot flashes are actually warm all the time. They tend to perspire easily, so they open a window because

Creepy-crawlies

In very rare cases, hot flashes can feel like insects crawling under and all over the skin, especially on the arms and scalp. Only a handful of women in my two decades of practicing women's health medicine have cited this feeling. They think they are going crazy when they feel a creepy-crawly sensation, which may be followed by typical hot flash symptoms. The best treatment for most women in this condition is hormone therapy, since these altered skin sensations may be related to drops in estrogen.

a room feels stuffy. They turn up the air-conditioning and then point to this menopause symptom as the culprit. "I'm having a hot flash!" they insist, when really they've just entered a room with a slightly elevated temperature that pushes them from warm to sweating.

If you're overheated all the time and you aren't flashing, you may have another reason for heat intolerance. Some very overweight women simply have too much insulation, as if they're wearing a winter coat in the summer.

There are other reasons unrelated to hormone changes that cause women to experience hot flashes. Many women with diabetes discover that the condition damages their autonomic nervous system, which is responsible for such bodily functions as perspiration and temperature regulation. People with over- or underactive thyroids may experience temperature fluctuations for similar reasons.

What Causes a Hot Flash?

You know what a hot flash feels like, but *why* does your body crank up the heat? Hot flashes are caused by hormone changes, particularly low and/or fluctuating estrogen levels, that occur during menopause.

Flash Versus Flush

When hot flashes also produce visible redness in the face and neck, they are called hot flushes. The "flush" refers to the redness itself.

Here's how it happens. A drop in estrogen signals the body's thermostat region, the hypothalamus in the brain. Until menopause, estrogen helps regulate the body's temperature, keeping it within its comfort zone and preventing us from overheating or breaking into sweats after small temperature shifts. But without the help of estrogen, some women become sensitive even to slight temperature changes that the rest of us don't notice.

As we lose estrogen before and during menopause, the brain says, "Uh-oh—it's getting hot in here." Reacting to the brain's message, the heart pumps faster, blood vessels in the skin dilate to circulate more blood and disperse the heat, and sweat glands gear up.

With the right level of estrogen, the brain's thermostat registers the message "The temperature is just fine." But some women's brain thermostats become overly sensitive as a result of hormone fluctuations and a drop in estrogen. There are also some nonhormonal factors that affect this sensitive thermostat, thereby adding to these disruptive hot flashes.

If your best friend isn't having hot flashes, then you may be wondering, "Why me?" Some women simply have more sensitive brain thermostats than others do. Other women in menopause may have just enough hormones to meet their body's needs, so their brains don't send warnings that something is out of balance. Like women who are prone to migraines, women who experience moderate to extreme hot flashes have brains that are programmed to be a bit more sensitive to changes and fluctuations.

An excess of weight can cause women to suffer
more from hot flashes—both in frequency and
severity—than they would if they were at a normal
weight. To combat this, some experts recommend
that even normal body weight women approaching
perimenopause and menopause work to lose five
to ten pounds prior to menopause to account for the
fact that many women gain five to fifteen pounds
during this life stage.

• • •

Heavier women, women who are under increased stress, and women who do not exercise regularly may have more intense hot flashes. That said, you can be slender, exercise daily, enjoy yoga and deep breathing, have a relatively stress-free life, and still have severe hot flashes. So while lifestyle changes and healthy living go a long way toward easing the transition into menopause, that's not enough for all women. It burns me up (no pun intended) when I meet women whose doctors have dismissed their complaints of hot flashes by telling them to exercise more or take a few deep breaths.

Just as doctors can treat migraines, we can treat hot flashes and with great results.

Causes and Triggers of Hot Flashes

Environmental triggers such as stress, stuffy rooms, or warm weather can set off your body temperature and cause hot flashes. Here are some other culprits:

- Caffeine
- Alcohol

- Spicy foods
- Tight clothing
- Heat
- Smoking cigarettes

Some women find they can control hot flashes by avoiding these triggers.

Tracking Your Triggers

To track down what specifically might be triggering your hot flashes, try recording when they occur and note any patterns. Carry a little spiral notebook with you for a few days and jot down what was going on just before the flash started.

Did you drink a cup of coffee? Did you have a glass of wine? Were you stressed out? Were you wearing tight clothes?

See whether there's a common theme and then work to eliminate that trigger.

To narrow the list of possible suspects, try recording when your hot flashes occur and note any patterns:

- Are you typically dealing with a stressful situation?
- Were you asleep?
- Do you notice that you flash immediately after eating a spicy dish?

If your episodes are mild to moderate, you can try these cool-down techniques:

- Wear layered clothing.
- Sip a cold drink.
- Arrive at meetings early so that you can choose a seat near a vent, window, or fan.

- If stress is a trigger, practice deep-breathing exercises to relax.
- Wear cotton, linen, and rayon clothing instead of synthetics, silk, or wool.
- Exercise daily.
- Stick your head in the freezer. It's a quick fix if you're at home or at the house of a good friend.

Night Sweats

Generally, hot flashes tend to be more severe at night, which is the worst time to get them. Not only are you hot and bothered, but you're losing sleep night after night. This compounds fatigue and affects mood, work performance, and overall health. (We'll talk more about ways to get a good night's sleep in chapter 8.)

For now, let's focus on timing. Why do you flash at night?

First, your body temperature normally dips a few notches as you sleep. This small decrease is a big deal if you lack estrogen. As your body temperature drops slightly, your brain says, "Time to turn on the heat—it's getting cold in here."

The result is a hot flash, which becomes a night sweat when your "cooling system" triggers the sweat glands into action. When you wake up hot and then wet, you eventually get cold.

Can I Prevent Night Sweats? Sleeping in a cool room with a fan and wearing socks can help you regulate body temperature while you sleep. Many women think that putting on socks will only make them hotter, but that's not the case. When you warm up peripheral extremities like hands and feet, your body temperature may be more stable. And when your body temperature is more stable, your brain doesn't send out errant messages to your body.

If night sweats are a problem, try these additional tips:

- Buy cotton sheets rather than synthetics.

- Wear natural fibers like cotton to bed.

- If your partner likes to sleep with layers of blankets, buy twin-sized covers for sleeping, so that you can both be comfortable.

- Lower the thermostat before you go to bed.

- Invest in a ceiling fan, air-conditioning, or even a handheld, battery-operated fan that you can flutter in front of your face if you wake up with a hot spell.

- Purchase a "chill pillow," which is a cooler pillow you can lay your head on or hug during a hot flash.

Treating Hot Flashes

Because menopausal symptoms can be bothersome to downright disruptive, there are several options for treatment.

Prescription Treatments

Short-term Hormone Therapy. A lack of estrogen and/or marked estrogen fluctuations can cause hot flashes. Replenishing a bit of the lost estrogen with HT works, plain and simple. In fact, I believe that estrogen is the most effective treatment for hot flashes.

Despite media assaults on hormone therapy, the fact is that the risks of low-dose treatment for a short term (less than 5–10 years) are minuscule for most healthy women who have recently become menopausal. The key is timing and periodic re-evaluation. There is no specific time limit to HT or to feeling well.

There's one chance in a thousand that you could suffer some consequence. This means that most women do very well on HT. They like the way their skin looks, their sex drive improves, they don't have dry vaginal tissues, their bone health improves, and yes, the hot flashes subside.

The NAMS website, *www.menopause.org,* posts updated statements on the use of estrogen and progestogens in peri- and postmenopausal women and classifies risks into rare and very rare categories. It also offers a very helpful compilation of the latest research into the benefits and risks of HT.

For the average woman with hot flashes, I might prescribe HT for two to three years until symptoms subside. When she is comfortable, I might reduce the estrogen dosage and wean her from hormone therapy, *if* that's what she wants and provided her sleep is good and her bones are stable. I have many women in my practice who have been on HT for years.

When hot flashes disrupt a woman's ability to function and participate in daily activities, as they did with Linda, I might suggest hormone therapy as a longer-term solution. For women who continue to have menopause symptoms when their HT is reduced or whose symptoms recur when they stop HT, I will also consider HT as a longer-term solution. In such cases, I insist on yearly exams and reassessments.

In the wake of the Women's Health Initiative (see page 161 in chapter 10 for a detailed explanation of this study and its effects on menopause treatment), women have been (inappropriately) told that all traditional prescription hormones are risky, so they have turned to alternatives, especially in the treatment of hot flashes. Women have been hoodwinked when they've been told that "natural bio-identical hormones compounded individually are safer and risk-free." Any hormone, including those hormones mixed on the premises by a compounding pharmacist, carries potential risks. [See Appendix 5: A Word on Compounding Pharmacies for a more detailed discussion of these risks and concerns.]

Antidepressants. As I noted previously, a handful of antidepressants are prescribed "off-label" for treatment of hot flashes. (*Off-*

Breast Cancer and Hot Flashes: Nonestrogen Options That Work

Some breast cancer treatments, particularly chemotherapy, can wipe out the ovaries, forcing some women into premature menopause. When that happens, estrogen levels drop suddenly, and hot flashes can be severe.

Hormone therapy isn't always appropriate for women with breast cancer or women taking the anti–breast cancer drug Tamoxifen (which has some estrogen-like effects) or aromatase inhibitors such as AROMASIN (exemestane), ARIMIDEX (anastrozole), and FEMARA (letrozole). This is when nonestrogen alternatives for treating menopause symptoms are important. For example, low doses of EFFEXOR XR (venlafaxine), an antidepressant, are often prescribed for hot flashes, as are some other nonprescription treatments.

PRISTIQ (desvenlafaxine) has been the first nonhormonal treatment for menopausal hot flashes specifically studied for rigorous hot flash reduction. PRISTIQ, approved as an antidepressant, has also shown particular benefit in treating hot flashes in women who are not depressed but who need hot flash control without the hormones.

PRISTIQ also has been shown to improve sleep in women—a big plus!

label means that the drug has been approved by the FDA for treating a disorder but not the one affecting you.)

These antidepressants have proven benefits for treating mood disorders and anxiety, but most have not been subjected to the same rigorous hot flash studies as hormone products. They may reduce the flashing, but they won't help a dry vagina, skin, or bone health. Furthermore, if you are a breast cancer survivor on Tamoxifen or taking Tamoxifen to reduce your risk of breast cancer, you should not take Paxil (paroxetine) to treat hot flashes as this SSRI has been shown to reduce Tamoxifen levels in some women by affecting the liver metabolism.

If a patient is not depressed but would rather be taking an antidepressant than hormone therapy, I prefer a low-dose SNRI (serotonin norepinephrine reuptake inhibitor), a class of antidepressants that includes the drug EFFEXOR XR.

EFFEXOR XR has an active isomer, desvenlafaxine, that is being studied in trials for depression, as well in trials of menopausal women who are not depressed but have disruptive hot flashes. And as mentioned earlier, under the brand name of PRISTIQ, it's likely to become the first nonhormonal medication approved by the FDA for the treatment of hot flashes.

Other Treatments. There are several other prescription treatments on the market for reducing hot flashes:

- **Megace (megestrol acetate).** A synthetic progestin that reduced hot flashes in a study of women with breast cancer. Its association with weight gain limits use in many menopausal women.

- **Catapres (clonidine).** A blood pressure drug sometimes prescribed to treat hot flashes in women with high blood pressure

- **Neurontin (gabapentin).** An antiseizure drug also used by some women for hot flashes. At high doses, it reduces hot flashes but can be associated with side effects such as dizziness and fluid retention.

Nonprescription Treatments

Herbal remedies. If you prefer a nonprescription approach to treating hot flashes, there are a few options. None of these is approved by the FDA, so you take a risk: we don't know what the long-term effects may be. In addition, a remedy for hot flashes is not necessarily a solution to all menopause-related health changes. In other words, taking black cohosh might reduce hot flashes, but it won't prevent bone loss or treat symptoms like vaginal dryness.

- **Black cohosh.** Some randomized trials suggest that the herb black cohosh is a short-term treatment for hot flashes and night sweats; however, black cohosh's effectiveness as a hot flash remedy is debatable. It may reduce sweating, but it will not necessarily treat all your menopause symptoms. Side effects include nausea and gastrointestinal upset.

  When a woman wants to try black cohosh, I recommend the over-the-counter brand Remifemin from Germany. The German Commission E (similar to our country's FDA) approves this form of black cohosh for use for up to six months to relieve hot flashes. Black cohosh and other herbs like valerian root have been associated with reports of liver toxicity, so long-term effects are a real concern.

- **Soy isoflavones.** Plant estrogens found in soy foods are thought to have weak estrogen-like effects. Choose soy foods rather than supplements and understand that not every woman's body converts soy isoflavones into the estrogen-like substance equol. (See the discussion in chapter 6 on page 106.)

- **Evening primrose oil.** Some women say this botanical reduces hot flashes, but there is no scientific evidence to support this. Side effects include nausea and diarrhea. Women with schizophrenia should not use evening primrose oil because it may worsen their condition.

- **Flaxseed.** This is certainly an important food to incorporate into your diet for the overall health benefits of omega-3 fats. Like soy foods, when it's used to replace animal fats,

Scrutinize So-Called Remedies

The brain is our most powerful organ, and if it believes a remedy is helping, it will help the body actually feel better. As the saying goes, mind over matter.

This is why researchers subject substances to placebo tests. One study group will be given the proposed remedy, and another group will be given an inert substance, or placebo. Researchers record how each group responds. Often, proposed treatments show no better results than their placebos because placebos are very powerful.

The power of suggestion is real. So when a woman says she took a special vitamin or concoction from a compounding pharmacy and it reduced her menopause symptoms, the question is whether the power of her own brain controlled her response or whether the remedy actually provided independent therapeutic effects.

The message: Choose remedies that have been subjected to placebo tests before making a choice about alternative medicines.

it may help lower cholesterol levels. Flaxseed is available in whole-seed and oil forms. (See on the discussion in chapter 6 on page 108.)

- **Vitamin E.** Taking 800 IU of vitamin E has been advocated to help hot flashes. A placebo-controlled, randomized study evaluated vitamin E supplements (800 IU/day for four weeks) for 120 breast cancer survivors with hot flashes and found that compared to the placebo, it decreased hot flashes slightly.

Alternative Treatments. Alternative remedies are a wise choice for women who have blood clots, women who have had breast cancer, or women who are taking Tamoxifen or undergoing other breast cancer treatments. In general, for these particular women, the risks of hormone therapy may outweigh taking even short-term HT.

Other women simply prefer nonprescription treatments or want to try those first. Just remember, you should always discuss even nonprescription drugs and vitamins with your doctor before taking them.

Chapter 8

Sleep: Difficulties and Disorders

S leep is one of the body's basic needs. It restores and preserves our health. Too little sleep puts us at risk for health problems such as high blood pressure and heart disease. When we are sleep deprived, immunity to sickness declines, and tolerance for stress plummets.

When we don't have a well-rested body and mind, every aspect of our waking day is affected. Yet statistics show that as many as 70 percent of Americans are sleep deprived.

Of course, some of those exhausted Americans are women in midlife. In fact, according to the National Sleep Foundation, women who report the most sleep problems are those in their perimenopause through postmenopause years. Their symptoms include hot flashes, mood disorders, insomnia, and sleep-disordered breathing. Such sleep problems are often accompanied by depression and anxiety.

Many women don't realize just how important sleep is, so they put it at the very bottom of the to-do list. We tend to squeeze every hour out of every day. We cram our schedules with professional, social, and family activities, rarely leaving time to relax and get to bed on time. But sleep is when the body renews and recharges itself with energy and strength for the next day.

Take Lawonda for instance.

Lawonda

Lawonda was so tired that she almost fell asleep at the wheel driving home. The night sweats that drenched her bed and hot flashes that jolted her from her sleep have taken their toll. She has gained weight since her period stopped and the snoring has gotten louder. She didn't even recognize this correlation because she has been so busy and so exhausted. It wasn't until I queried her about her specific sleep pattern that she realized there might be a relationship between menopause, fatigue, weight gain, and sleep problems.

Lawonda had both a menopausal-related sleep disorder from hot flashes, which were well controlled on an estrogen/progesterone combination, as well as a primary sleep disorder, obstructive sleep apnea syndrome. After being fitted for a nasal CPAP device, a small portable electronic device that gives continuous positive pressure to the upper airway, her snoring stopped, her sleep improved and with a combination of hormone therapy, her disruptive hot flashes and drenching night sweats stopped. In her case, I selected PROMETRIUM, or natural micronized progesterone. Natural progesterone is a mild respiratory stimulant and, in many women, causes some mild sedation as natural progesterone is converted to a natural sedative hypnotic.

When I saw Lawonda back in the office two months later, she had dropped ten pounds, felt so much more energetic, and was not having trouble remembering activities. She told me on a recent business trip, when she was at the airport, she had noticed three other people checking in their portable CPAP machines.

Sleep Problems

When your head finally hits the pillow at the end of the day, your mind is probably still racing, and your inner dialogue may sound something like this:

> *I'm so tired. How come I can't relax? I've got to get to sleep—I have a million things to do tomorrow. I've got to fin- ish that report and get Mom to her doctor's appointment. And I can't remember, does Jessie need a ride home after soccer prac- tice? I can't keep up. I'm just not feeling right these days. Oh, I hope I don't have hot flashes tonight.*

If you have trouble falling or staying asleep, you may have a problem that needs medical attention. During midlife, it's impor- tant to sort out whether a sleep problem is related to menopause symptoms or if it's a "primary" sleep disorder—a condition that creates sleep problems but has nothing to do with menopause.

Is Menopause Causing My Sleep Problems?

Menopause itself doesn't cause difficulty sleeping, but its symptoms certainly can. As we've discussed, hot flashes occur more frequently at night, causing interrupted sleep and tiredness the next day. In addition, our daily stresses and concerns with the physical changes we're experiencing tend to "turn on" when the lights go off. Our minds go into overdrive, and we ruminate.

Menopause-related anxiety, depression, and mood swings can keep thoughts churning long past bedtime. For some women, the physical and psychological changes they experience during the menopause years can feel like a bad dream that won't go away.

Here's a hopeful note. Although we can't treat sleep problems with hormone therapy, we can use it to treat menopause symptoms that deprive you of the rest you need. Often, restoring hormone balance with low-dose, short-term hormone therapy will help you get a good night's sleep. Women who prefer not to take hormone therapy can discuss alternative options, but if the cause of the sleep disturbance is menopausal symptoms, then the sleep problem is best treated with HT. Alternatively, antidepressants like PRISTIQ can be used and may help improve sleep. And if you have a primary sleep problem, there are many excellent treatments available today.

But before you can rest easy, you and your doctor will need to figure out whether your symptoms are related to menopause or a sleep disorder.

What Qualifies as a "Sleep Problem?"

Whether related to menopause or not, sleep problems show up in a number of different ways, which may include the following:

- Trouble falling asleep
- Difficulty staying asleep
- Waking too early and being unable to get back to sleep
- Finding it hard to wake up on time
- Being tired during the day
- Sleeping too much

What Can I Do About It?

If you are experiencing one or more of the following difficulties and are in midlife, your sleep problems might be an indication of a menopause-related symptom.

Hot Flashes and Night Sweats. Depending on how severe your hot flashes are, you may benefit from alternative remedies (discussed in chapter 7) or hormone therapy. Otherwise, try these tips to keep cool at night:

- Wear loose clothing to bed.
- Keep your bedroom cool and well ventilated.
- Avoid taking hot showers or baths before bed.
- Sleep with your socks on to help regulate body temperature.

Physical Discomfort. Menopause symptoms that can set you up for a poor night's sleep include hot flashes, itchy skin, a dry vagina—any physical irritation that is bothering you.

If you had a pounding headache, you'd probably take a pain reliever to alleviate it. Why wouldn't you treat menopause symptoms so that you can rest at night? Use the various treatments discussed throughout this book to care for your symptoms, and sleep is likely to come much more easily.

Mood Swings, Depression, or Anxiety. Natural ways to improve your mood include eating right, exercising regularly, and practicing relaxation techniques to restore balance.

You can also try taking vitamin B, which is believed to boost mood because it restores elements involved in different aspects of brain chemistry. (See chapter 4 for more details.)

If you remain depressed or anxious for more than two weeks, it's important to see a doctor. Only a physician can properly determine whether your case calls for a prescription to treat depression or anxiety.

Stress. Most of us don't have an "off button" that allows us to erase the day's stressors when we retire at night. Instead, thoughts of

Is Bedtime the Right Time for Your Medicine?

I advise many of my patients to take their hormone therapy medication at night. This makes sense because the dose lasts through their sleeping hours, making it less likely that menopausal symptoms, including hot flashes, will wake them.

family, work, and personal affairs churn in our heads as soon as we turn off the lights. We lie in bed and worry and think.

Relaxation techniques are an important part of slowing down at the end of the day. Establish a bedtime ritual like taking a warm bath, reading a favorite book, or writing in a journal to set the mood for sleep. Consider the hour before your bedtime as "you time."

• • • *Fast Fact* • • •

Some women find that taking a magnesium supplement at bedtime helps induce sleep. In a happy menopause two-for-one deal, magnesium also reduces the constipation that is a side effect of taking calcium supplements.

• • •

Drowsy Days Can Drag You Down, Too

How you feel during the day is just as important as how many times you wake up at night. Daytime fatigue means that your body isn't getting the rest it needs to function.

Don't justify daytime drowsiness as "payback" for running too many errands, being too programmed, or having too much work to do. You can't expect to live life to its fullest if you aren't sleeping at night.

Tune into these daytime warning signs:

- Are you tired or lagging most days, despite a good night's sleep?

- Do you rely on caffeine to get you through the day?

- Do you notice a shortened attention span?

- Do you feel unmotivated or lack the energy to "get going?"

- Do you fall asleep during meetings?

- Do you notice a decline in work performance, reluctance to participate in family activities you once enjoyed, or neglect of certain hobbies because you're "just too tired?"

Try the tips below, what doctors call good "sleep hygiene," to stop sleep problems in their tracks:

- Reserve your bedroom for sleep and intimacy. If you have trouble sleeping, don't use it for activities like watching television or reading.

- Sleep only when you're drowsy.

- If you cannot fall or stay asleep, leave your bedroom and read or engage in a relaxing activity in another room.

- Maintain regular times for going to bed and getting up.

- Avoid napping during the day. (If you're extremely exhausted, limit naps to less than one hour, and don't nap after 3 PM)

- Avoid strenuous exercise within six hours of going to sleep.

Snoring: A Warning Sign of Serious Illness

If you are very tired during the day, you may be waking up at night without realizing it. People with obstructive sleep apnea wake up at night because they stop breathing, then immediately fall asleep again. In the morning, they are unaware that their sleep has been disturbed many times throughout the night. They are puzzled as to why they feel so tired.

Usually, their bed partner is not so puzzled, having heard the snore-choke-stop-gasp breathing pattern all night long.

If you snore at night and are sleepy during the day, let your doctor know. When untreated, sleep apnea can result in dangerous complications, including cardiovascular problems.

- Minimize light, noise, and extreme temperatures in the bedroom.
- Practice healthy eating. Avoid large meals before bedtime. Stay away from spicy foods that may trigger hot flashes.
- Avoid nicotine, caffeine, and alcohol before bedtime.
- Dress in lightweight clothes that "breathe" (cotton and natural fibers).
- Use a fan or air-conditioning to cool the room.
- Practice relaxation techniques such as massage, meditation, and exercise to reduce stress.
- If you feel depressed or anxious, talk to a doctor or behavioral health professional.

When Do I Need to See a Doctor?

If any kind of sleep-related problem is bothering you, schedule an appointment with your doctor. Only a physician can determine whether hormone therapy is appropriate for your situation or whether you require a consultation with a sleep specialist.

Practice "Investigative Journalism." I recommend starting a sleep journal before you go to your appointment. Recording the following information will help your physician help you:

- What time do you go to bed at night and wake up each morning?
- How many times do you wake during the night?
- Do you fall asleep again quickly after waking?
- How many minutes/hours do you stay awake during the night?
- What is your caffeine, alcohol, nicotine, and food intake before bedtime?
- Are there any environmental disruptions that cause awakenings (noisy neighbors, an uncomfortably hot room, too much light)?

Some women may turn to over-the-counter aids such as Tylenol PM, and occasional use is fine. I do not recommend melatonin bought over the counter since no pure, "pharmaceutical-grade" product is currently available.

The melatonin receptor agent Rozerem (ramelteon) is a new prescription medication without addictive potential. It is worth considering if you have tried good sleep hygiene and made lifestyle changes, but still have trouble sleeping.

A number of other prescription sleeping pills, such as Ambien CR (zolpidem tartrate) and Lunesta (eszopiclone), can be taken long-term. However, they may have addictive potential and must be carefully monitored.

What If It Is a Sleep Disorder?

Forty million Americans have sleep disorders, according to the American Academy of Sleep Medicine, so don't assume that any sleeping problems you have are necessarily related to menopause.

If you answer yes to any of the following questions, ask your doctor if you should be tested for a sleep disorder:

- Are you often tired or sleepy during the day?
- Do you snore or have interrupted breathing during sleep?
- Do you kick or thrash in your sleep?
- Do you have trouble falling or staying asleep?
- Do you have a family history of sleep disorders?
- Do you have unusual sensations in your legs at night that interfere with your ability to fall asleep?
- Do you experience unusual behaviors in sleep, such as walking, eating, or acting out dreams?
- Do you have irregular or inconsistent sleep and wake-up times? Is your bedroom environment noisy, bright, or uncomfortable?

Your doctor should give you a sleep questionnaire and perform a physical exam and may refer you to a sleep center to see a specialist. (It's a good idea to be sure that the facility is licensed by the American Academy of Sleep Medicine. You can log on to *www. sleepeducation.com* for information.)

The sleep professionals may conduct an overnight evaluation, or "sleep study," during which you will be hooked up to various monitors that record breathing, heart rate, and brain waves while you sleep. Treatments depend on diagnoses, which can vary widely. *The International Classification of Sleep Disorders,* second edition, documents eighty-one official sleep disorders.

Chapter 9

Menopause and Sex

Not in the mood? You may be wondering, *Is it hormones? Is it my partner? Or is this lack of interest due to normal aging?* Lack of sex drive is very common in women, and a complete assessment is needed if you have a change in sexual function that is distressing to you. When sex is painful, this is a "red flag" that there could be a hormonal deficiency.

Melissa

Once my ovaries were gone after the hysterectomy, so were my libido and my sex life. I knew my hysterectomy was going to fast-forward my body into menopause and all the physical changes that go along with it. And because my estrogen level would drop dramatically following the surgical procedure, I mentally prepared myself for hot flashes. But I had no idea that my hysterectomy also would create a Continental Divide in my bed, with my husband on one side and me on the other. He was sympathetic but frustrated and concerned because he couldn't work his old magic. I was frustrated, too—and in quite a bit of pain. I was feeling like sandpaper down there, rather than like a woman ready to make a move.

I tried everything. I relaxed with a glass of red wine, flipped off the lights, and turned on the charm, but I soon just gave up on sex. It hurt too much!

My insensitive surgeon suggested buying erotic videotapes and scouring the "sexy" aisle in the nearest lingerie shop to rev up my sex life. But as I quickly learned, erotica cannot make a thin, painful vagina healthy.

Different Perspectives on Sex

It should come as no surprise that women think differently from men about sex. Our emotions toy with our brains and send mixed signals to our bodies. If we're unhappy in our relationships, stressed out at work, or just feeling "blah" because of all those hot flashes and a few extra pounds, our brains will say, "Nope. No sex tonight." And our bodies will respond, "No way, no how."

But men come home from a long day at work and look at sex as stress release. If everything has gone wrong, the one thing that can make it right is . . . you guessed it: sex. The brain gives a direct order to the body, "I want sex." And boom, he's ready. Emotions aren't always a factor.

Imagine the frustration that results from this biological mismatch.

Faced with their different perspectives, a couple often will have difficulty getting into the moment. Gradually, the moments pass, and pass.

When I talk to my patients, I often discover this gap between the expectations of men and women, as well as a lack of open discussion about sex. Many times, sexual dysfunction in a relationship has nothing to do with menopause. But how do you know?

This chapter will address some of the most common complaints and concerns about sex that midlife women face, examining how they may be affected by the onset of menopause. We'll also discuss other possible factors that you can address with your partner and your doctor.

Sex and Intimacy Changes

If you rate your sex life as unsatisfactory or even unpleasant, you're not alone. Up to 40 percent of women experience sexual dysfunction at some point in their lives, and women who have had their ovaries removed at an early age may be the most affected. Difficulties can range from basic lack of desire to painful sexual activity.

Every woman responds to sex and intimacy in an individual way. In fact, changes in sexual function are not considered medical problems unless they're causing you distress or pain. Many women are content with a sexual slowdown around midlife. What's more, hormones are not always to blame for sexual problems.

Still, menopause can introduce physical changes that interrupt a happy sex life. For example, estrogen loss causes thinning of the vaginal tissue, which becomes dry and more susceptible to irritation and bleeding.

Other common sexual complaints associated with menopause include these:

- Slower sexual arousal
- Less lubrication during sex
- Sensitive skin in the vaginal area
- Painful intercourse

For women who undergo hysterectomies, a dramatic decrease in estrogen exacerbates menopausal symptoms. One in six women experiences significant changes following a hysterectomy, and most of those who report severe menopause-related problems had complete procedures (removal of the uterus and ovaries).

Even when only the uterus is removed, the clamping of blood vessels during the procedure can reduce blood flow to the ovaries and affect their production of hormones.

All this means that talking with your doctor is critical if you plan to continue to enjoy sexual intimacy throughout menopause and beyond. Start by describing the problem. Then your physician can help you determine whether your solution is HT, sex therapy, or introducing a bit of spice to tired bedroom habits.

Be open with your physician. If he or she doesn't ask you about your sex life, you need to raise the subject, volunteer information, and ask questions. Sex is an integral part of our relationships and our personal health. Don't tag it as an X-rated subject or discount its importance to your overall happiness. And particularly if you are frustrated or in pain, do not keep silent.

Risks of Postmenopausal Sex

Wanting to have sex is generally a sign of good health in that any mental or physical ailment usually zaps drive. Sexual activity requires some exertion, and physical activity is good for your health! That said, sex can still be dangerous if you put yourself at risk for STIs (sexually transmitted infections). I've seen many midlife women and even great-grandmother geriatric women, freed from the burden of pregnancy concerns, throw caution to the wind and end up with serious infections. While not life threatening, many STIs, like genital herpes and genital warts, can be painful and very embarrassing. But some STIs *are* life threatening, the most serious one being HIV (human immunodeficiency virus). *Any* exchange of any bodily fluid can put you at risk. Mutual monogamy with a trusted partner and "safer sex" techniques like the consistent use of a latex condom must be given high priority. And sex toys should be cleaned and not shared.

Isn't It Natural for Sex to Become Less Enjoyable as You Age?

If you think that enduring uncomfortable sex is just a part of getting older, it's time to retrain your thoughts. You should be able to enjoy sex as long as you can eat and breathe. Even on your 85th birthday, if you like.

Of course, our feelings about sex and our bodies will change as we age, but our mechanisms should still be primed for the job. So then we need to ask whether the root of our sexual dissatisfaction is physical, psychological, or both. Are hormone changes responsible for sexual dysfunction, or are underlying issues inhibiting the necessary brain-body connections that trigger sexual pleasure?

If the answer were simple, all women would be having great sex.

Key Sexual Concerns at Midlife

The key sexual issues women face in midlife are the following:

- Low sex drive
- Arousal disorder
- Painful sex: atrophic vaginitis

Low Sex Drive

Lack of sex drive tops the list of sexual frustrations that women experience during midlife. So many of them come to me and say something like, "I don't feel sexy. I have too much on my mind. I'm never in the mood. I used to be interested all the time. What happened?"

Many women who report low sex drive still want to have physical intimacy with their partners, and many of them also say that they have previously been active in the bedroom, just not lately.

Sex drive naturally decreases as we age. The energy we had in our 20s and 30s—the reproduction years—declines. Our biological clocks reflect the fact that we no longer need to procreate. Women's lives are divided into cycles, and when the baby-making stage ends and menopause begins, sex drive changes accordingly.

A decreased sex drive during menopause isn't necessarily a problem for every woman. Some women accept a lower sex drive and are happy with less sex, preferring to express their love in other ways. (Many men share this preference for noncoital intimacy.) Some women never really enjoyed sex to begin with; this is a matter of preference and completely normal. In such cases, low sex drive is *not* a medical concern.

On the other end of the spectrum, once they have no worries about pregnancy, no children at home to dampen the mood, and fewer stresses in life and work—all of which are normally obstacles to stoking the fires—some women notice an increased sex drive during menopause years. More comfortable in their bodies, these women embrace their midlife sexuality.

On the assumption that your bedroom nightlife doesn't fit this description, let's explore the topic a bit more. A good question to ask yourself is whether or not you're having an enjoyable sexual relationship with someone other than your partner.

This question may surprise you. But I have counseled many women who complain that they have no sex drive, that they are not attracted to their partners, and that they are unable to reach climax. Assuming that such a patient is distressed by the situation, I ask her, "Are you attracted to your partner?" If the answer is no, the sexual dysfunction is not a medical or menopausal issue; it's a relationship problem. Because it's important for me to know a patient's sexual history for reasons of disease prevention and to provide general health advice, I always ask whether the woman has more than one partner. Sometimes a woman says yes. She's having an affair and feels like a 25-year-old sex goddess while she's with another man, yet has no sexual chemistry with her husband. She wonders why her husband can't turn her on.

In such a case, the "treatment" involves treating the relationship. The best way to do this is for the couple to enter therapy with a professional who is trained and skilled in counseling couples.

Finding Lost Libido. Let's assume that you're still attracted to your partner and want to maintain a sexually intimate relationship. It may be instructive to take a look at the anatomy of libido.

Hormones and their proper balance play a significant role in sex drive. Although testosterone gets credited with being the "king" of sex hormones, estrogen is the "queen" of female sexuality.

During menopause, your estrogen-testosterone balance may be off-kilter, and when estrogen isn't playing its part, you feel it. Your vaginal area is thin, weak, and dry and won't lubricate during foreplay. When the vagina isn't physically prepared for intercourse, the act is quite painful. Also, spontaneous desire or the unprovoked urge to have sex may naturally lessen for many women who are past the age of reproduction.

Actually, during menopause, our male partners often have more estrogen than we do. Their testicles still produce testosterone, which gets converted into estrogen, while our own estrogen sources disappear and production slows.

The best way for some women to boost libido lost when removal of the ovaries abruptly brings about hormone imbalance (as in Melissa's case) is to restore what's been taken away.

Lately, women have been asking me to prescribe testosterone, having heard that replenishing lost stores of this sex hormone will prime them for a better nightlife. But testosterone is usually not a stand-alone solution for women who suffer from menopause-related low libido. Estrogen and testosterone work together, so filling up on testosterone alone won't help unless your estrogen status is adequate. Having a hormonal imbalance with too much testosterone can cause acne, mood symptoms, abnormal hair growth, abnormal hair loss, deepening of the voice, and an elevated blood count, so women on testosterone therapies need to be monitored closely.

That said, a testosterone patch (awaiting FDA approval pending more long-term studies) could change the way we treat both premenopausal and postmenopausal female sexual dysfunction. We would finally be able to treat women who have sexual problems with a standardized dose of testosterone.

The testosterone patch, Intrinsa, is already available in Europe by prescription. It is a shame that American women do not yet have this option.

Currently, for the most part, we are forced to give women much smaller doses of testosterone products formulated for men or have compounding pharmacies mix up testosterone. At this time, one estrogen-testosterone pill combination, Estratest HS, has been given to women who are dealing with treatment-resistant hot flashes. It is also being studied for its effects on sexual function. There are testosterone gels, such as LibiGel, in clinical studies. Off-label medicines currently used for erectile dysfunction in men (like Viagra, Cialis, and Levitra) have sometimes been used in women with genital arousal problems and women with orgasmic dysfunction caused by antidepressants (we'll discuss antidepressants and sex in a moment).

For certain women, I will write prescriptions for testosterone compounded in gel forms. However, this type of treatment must usually be balanced with estrogen therapy.

I'd like to emphasize that while women can find testosterone at compounding pharmacies, the formulas obtained from these pharmacies are not regulated by the FDA. Please remember my earlier warning that just because you get a treatment from a compounding pharmacy doesn't mean that it is effective and safe. Too much testosterone can wreak havoc on your skin (acne) and result in thinning of hair, growth of hair in unwanted places, or both.

There are other ways to rev up libido:

- If you enjoy an occasional alcoholic beverage, have a glass of wine with dinner two to three times a week. Alcohol taken in moderation may boost hormone levels. (Make it red wine, and you'll also be getting important antioxidants into your diet.)

- Don't overeat in the evening. Large meals can sabotage any after-dinner romance if you're feeling stuffed and ready to snooze.

- Exercise on a regular basis. It's no secret that endorphins—the "feel-good" hormones—can spark desire. Exercise combined with time to relax and focus on yourself is a wonderful aphrodisiac.

If you are having sex with a male and are not worried about pregnancy and/or sexually transmitted infections, then direct vaginal mucosal contact with his semen/ejaculated fluid (which contains sperm, prostaglandins, prostatic secretions, and testosterone) can be an aphrodisiac for many women.

Arousal Disorder

The next question to ask yourself when your love life has stalled is whether or not you get aroused when you think about sex.

Your answer is crucial, because arousal and sex drive are two different things. If you desire sex and are in the mood for it but your vaginal zone will not respond by lubricating and preparing for intercourse, then what you're suffering from is an arousal disorder, defined as the inability to achieve or maintain a state of arousal. An arousal disorder can occur at the brain level and/or the genital level. But don't automatically blame menopause. The lack of arousal may be due to any of the following:

- Certain high blood pressure medications
- Heart disease and diabetes
- Antidepressant therapies, particularly SSRIs

- Past pelvic surgery (including hysterectomy, traumatic childbirth, or a bladder lift), which can damage nerves in the vaginal zone

If you and your doctor rule out these possibilities, it's time to look at your hormonal status. As we noted, estrogen is responsible for physically preparing your body for intercourse. But during menopause, estrogen levels are low, a condition that especially affects "female" areas needing estrogen to function.

Because estrogen loss makes vaginal tissues fragile and collagen loss reduces pelvic elasticity, the genitals may not get very "revved up" for sex. And because the dry, thin tissue can be uncomfortable, the brain is also sending messages warning, "This will not be comfortable!" Furthermore, we live in the Viagra era; older men with erectile difficulties are using pharmaceuticals to maintain firmer erections that may produce further discomfort for women whose genitalia are already fragile.

Lack of response to sexual advances can diminish a sexual relationship between a man and woman over time. If your partner is

Sex and Antidepressants

If a woman has untreated depression and is suffering from the resulting fatigue, low mood, poor concentration, and anhedonia (lack of pleasure in previously pleasurable activities), then it is no mystery why she would not have a sex drive. Many times treating depression improves all of these symptoms. Conversely, women who are not depressed or suffering from sexual dysfunction and are prescribed higher-dose SSRI antidepressants to treat their hot flashes ironically *develop* female sexual dysfunction (FSD). This is one reason why I favor using lower-dose NSRIs to treat hot flashes if a woman cannot or will not take HT.

erect and your body is unwilling to respond, his excitement will diminish when he can't please you. Also, because it may be more difficult for you to have sex when your tissues are dry and fragile, you probably won't be interested in what quickly becomes a painful act. (We'll talk more about this in chapter 11.) This downward spiral can occur over several years.

• • • *Fast Fact* • • •

Testosterone gets the credit for triggering sexual thoughts and fantasies—for initiating spontaneous sex drive. However, it is estrogen that keeps the vagina healthy.

• • •

Hormone Therapy for Arousal. The best way to treat a genital-arousal disorder in a woman is to replenish estrogen, at least locally, meaning in the vagina. Without this hormone, you cannot achieve the physical response necessary to have comfortable, enjoyable vaginal intercourse. As with any hormone therapy, your doctor should be able to advise you regarding what type (cream, pill, vaginal ring) is most appropriate. Remember, you have a choice.

I recommend local estrogen therapy to treat vaginal atrophy, dryness, and sexual dysfunction in many of my patients. Most of them happily report that it works.

Treating Dryness. You can also purchase over-the-counter products to lubricate the vaginal area. Water-soluble ointments such as K-Y Jelly and Astroglide are best; they won't weaken latex condoms the way mineral oil or Vaseline will. (You should avoid using both of these in the vagina.)

Be aware that these lubricants are usually a quick fix, though. You're treating dryness only. Women who choose to use them should also consider using a vaginal moisturizer (such as Replens or Silk-E) a few times a week, rather than only before having sex. For a combination vaginal moisturizer and lubricant, you can use vitamin E oil or olive oil.

Why Viagra Is Usually Just for Men. Men may have trouble keeping the penis engorged, and much of male sexual dysfunction is related to erectile problems. Women don't usually have the sexual equivalent of this problem (with the exception of women who have diabetes, pelvic nerve damage, or spinal cord injuries).

Women's problems with sexual function are very different from men's, and they have no quick fix comparable to Viagra. For most women, the most important sex organ is actually the brain, and arousal problems start there. Estrogen primes the brain for sex, testosterone initiates desire, and then estrogen helps the genitalia respond to sexual stimulation.

Painful Sex: Atrophic Vaginitis

When vaginal tissue becomes fragile, brittle, dry, and irritated, the condition is referred to as vaginal atrophy. Some women sarcastically joke that they are "drying up." In fact, that's what happens.

For women who suffer from vaginal atrophy, intercourse is very painful. They might experience friction burns while having sex, their skin tightens—making the act even more uncomfortable—and bleeding can occur. Sex is no longer appealing, understandably so.

Consider your reaction to a food that once made you sick, perhaps from an allergic reaction or food poisoning. If you even see the food again, you may begin to feel queasy. Your body is trying to protect you from further illness or injury. The same goes for sex. Your libido and sex drive drop because your brain associates sex with pain or injury. Not only are you physically unprepared for intercourse, you're not interested.

The frustration of feeling turned off by sex with their partners when they previously enjoyed it makes vaginal atrophy a distressing situation for many women. It's certainly a cause for medical attention. Fortunately, it's easily treated. Unfortunately, many women I see in my practice have never been offered the simple solutions that not only improve the health of the vagina but also have been shown to reduce the risk of recurrent bladder infections.

Lubricants aren't enough to treat an atrophic vaginal area. Because a thin vagina indicates extremely low estrogen levels, vaginal and/or systemic hormone therapy is the best bet.

Hormone Therapy Options for Atrophic Vaginitis.

- **Vaginal ring (ESTRING or FEMRING).** A flexible ring inserted into the vagina releases hormones at a steady rate and is especially helpful for improving skin texture in the vaginal zone. Rings generally must be replaced every three months. (The Femring releases higher doses of estrogen than the Estring, so it affects the entire body instead of just the vagina and bladder.) The Estring is a good option for women who cannot use systemic, full-body hormone therapy, such as breast cancer patients and/or women with blood clots.

- **Vaginal estrogen creams (ESTRACE or PREMARIN).** Spread these on the genitals and insert into the vagina (with an applicator, or, in severe cases of vaginal thinning and narrowing, with fingers).

- **Vaginal tablet (VAGIFEM).** This tiny pill is inserted into the lower third of the vagina twice a week (either with a finger or with the enclosed applicator). The pill releases small amounts of estrogen. Even lower doses of Vagifem have been found to be beneficial—I offer vaginal estrogen therapy to virtually every woman I examine who has any evidence of thinning and atrophy. Every woman deserves to have a healthy vagina!

Nonhormonal Options. These treatments, though not proven, show results in some women. Talk to your doctor before trying them to find out whether these options are suitable for you:

- **Silk-E or Replens.** As mentioned earlier, these nonhormonal vaginal moisturizers can be used a few times a week.

- **Vitamin E or olive oil.** A few times a week, these can be applied directly to the vagina and external genitalia to soothe the area. Many of my patients are surprised when I tell them they can use olive oil on their genitals. A few have smiled and asked me, "Extra virgin olive oil?"

Spice It Up

Brain-imaging equipment makes passion visible; you can actually see the excitement in someone who has a new partner. This fire has nothing to do with age. An 80-year-old person with a new partner may be more sexually active than a 50-year-old who has just celebrated a 25th wedding anniversary. While you probably can't capture the intensity of a six-month relationship (when partners are intoxicated by mutual discovery), you and your partner can certainly turn up the action in your bedroom if you're feeling stale.

Here are some suggestions for improving intimacy:

- Educate yourself about age-related sexual changes so that you can overcome anxiety about sexual function and performance.

- Try using erotic materials (videos or books) and change your sexual routines.

- Change your environment. Get away for a night or even a few hours.

- Practice relaxation techniques. Give each other massages or unwind with deep breathing to release stress and get in the moment.

- Increase communication and comfort with your partner through noncoital activities (physically stimulating behavior that does not include intercourse).

- Minimize pain by using sexual positions that allow you to control penetration.

- Practice Kegel exercises to strengthen pelvic muscles, improve elasticity, and enhance pleasure during intercourse. Contract the pelvic muscles for three seconds, then release. Do this 20 to 25 times at least once each day.

- Some women report increased genital sensation with Zestra (a mix of botanical oils and extracts) or topical arginine, both of which can be obtained over the counter at drug stores. Whether there is true effect on genital blood flow and nerve sensation beyond the positive placebo response of rubbing something on to the genitals has yet to be determined.

- Plan a romantic evening. Make a weekly date with your partner and take turns choosing a place to eat or visit. Let this be time you look forward to spending together.

Hitting the Right Spot

Finally, if you don't know already, find out where your erogenous zones are and be sure to share this information with your partner!

For many women, the most sensitive erogenous zone is the clitoris, and they need direct stimulation of this area. Many normal women are only able to climax with direct (hand, mouth, and/or vibrator) stimulation of the clitoris. Women are reassured when I tell them this is normal, for many erroneously believe that only the vagina is erogenous and that they are only supposed to have "vaginal orgasms." For other women, the most sensitive erogenous zone is the G-spot, located midway up on the anterior vaginal way (just behind the urethra). These women can usually climax with penile-vaginal intercourse. And for some, the key to climax is simultaneous stimulation of the entire vagina, G-spot, and the clitoris, a combination dubbed the "cligva" by sex therapists.

A very small percent of women report sexual satisfaction with direct cervical tapping—stimulation to the cervix, which is at the apex/top of the vagina. Also reported is satisfaction with nipple and breast stimulation and even anal intercourse, which can indirectly stimulate the G-spot.

Not all women are "wired" the same way. What causes pleasure in one woman might cause pain or discomfort in another one. Sometimes the response of different erogenous zones can change with age and with pregnancy. On a positive note, since sexual satisfaction is complex and dynamic in women and not one simple on or off switch, many women retain sexual function and sexual capacity even with various medical, hormonal, surgical, and radiation therapies, in contrast to many men who undergo prostate surgery or radiation and lose the capacity to maintain an erection.

More research is needed on female sexual function and female sexual dysfunction (FSD) to find simpler, more universal treatments. But for now, there does not appear to be any one truly universal aphrodisiac better than an attractive, respectful, loving partner!

Chapter 10

The Risks and Benefits of Hormone Therapy

Hormone therapy is still the best treatment available for menopausal symptoms, and the case is far from closed regarding its effects on other medical conditions (blood pressure, heart disease, colon cancer, Alzheimer's disease, major depression, Parkinson's disease, arthritis, and the eye condition macular degeneration). Furthermore, lower doses of hormones than previously studied may well provide the same benefits while reducing side effects. The use of progestogens (progestins and progesterone) may be the part of the equation that increases risk for breast cancer while protecting the uterus. Using estrogen transdermally, as in a weekly patch like Climara Pro or a daily estrogen lotion or gel, may reduce the risk of blood clots, but it may not raise the HDL-cholesterol as well as oral estrogen.

In short, we need more research. But in the meantime, there are more options for treating menopause symptoms than ever before. This should be the best time for midlife women—but instead, many suffer needlessly. Take Anne Marie for instance.

Anne Marie

I didn't know what to believe. One study said not to take any hormones. Another said that estrogen use by older women could increase their risk of stroke. Every day there was a new headline with a different warning. You'd think I'd been treating my menopausal symptoms with illegal narcotics!

I took PREMPRO for several years without a problem before discovering that I was risking my life—at least, according to the media reports. My doctor suggested that I taper down the dosage, but I insisted on cutting it out completely. So I quit cold turkey.

The result of my rash decision was disastrous. I felt as if someone had pulled the rug out from under me. I was anxious and extremely uncomfortable all the time. My hot flashes were so severe that I sometimes wondered whether I could leave the house to run errands. I never realized how much hormone therapy had been helping until I quit.

I tried some alternatives—black cohosh for hot flashes, vitamin E for vaginal discomfort. Nothing worked as well as my original treatment. To add insult to injury, I lost an inch in height and found out that my bones were thinning.

With so many misleading reports about what's good for women today, it seems as if just breathing is a risk. But I decided that I had to feel comfortable. I went back on hormone therapy—low-dose PREMPRO—and I finally feel normal again.

Taking Hormone Therapy

Millions of women have done well on hormone therapy, finding relief from the worst of their symptoms without increasing any other health risks. Remember, hormone therapy was and still is the only FDA-approved treatment for symptoms of menopause, including treatment of vaginal atrophy and the management of postmenopausal osteoporosis. And the FDA and most physicians regard all hormones as having potential benefits as well as potential risks, though these unfortunately get overshadowed by fearful media hype.

Where Do All These Misconceptions and Fears Come From?

The Women's Health Initiative (WHI) was a large, randomized trial that changed the way women—as well as much of the medical community—view HT. This change was not for the better. Fear, anxiety, and fewer choices for women resulted from misinterpretation of the sections of the study that focused on hormone therapy. Ironically, these studies had been initially designed to help women better understand the risks and benefits of HT.

Now the media, our friends, and even some of our doctors are inappropriately waving accusatory fingers at hormone therapy as a treatment for menopausal symptoms. This should infuriate women and spark a new debate that asks some very pointed questions about the treatment of women in modern America. For example, we might wonder:

- How accurate are randomized studies when applied to different groups of women for different reasons?
- Why have the media scared women into thinking they do not have choices, and why have otherwise good doctors also misinterpreted these studies?

- What about quality of life and sexual function for midlife women?
- How can women fairly assess what hormone therapy truly represents for their individual cases?

In this chapter, I will discuss the facts that women absolutely must know. These are details you probably won't read in the newspaper, because many articles for the lay public just skim the surface. There's far too much at stake with your health for research to be interpreted in such a superficial way.

Millions of women have done well on hormone therapy, finding relief from the worst of their symptoms without increasing any other health risks.

The FDA and most physicians regard all hormones as having potential benefits as well as potential risks just like with any prescription medicine.

Women's Health Initiative: The Hard Facts. In 2002, researchers halted part of the Women's Health Initiative. This was a preventive study funded by the National Institutes of Health (NIH) to focus on strategies for preventing heart disease, breast and colorectal cancer, and osteoporosis in postmenopausal women. A fifteen-year, multimillion-dollar project, the WHI involved 161,808 women ranging in age from 50 to 79.

The segment of the study that was halted had been assessing the long-term use of hormone therapy as a prevention tool for chronic illnesses because a preventive agent can essentially have no side effects. It is important to understand this was *not* a menopausal treatment trial.

Early information indicated that women who were postmenopausal and using PREMPRO (a combination of estrogen and progestin) faced a slightly increased risk of being diagnosed with breast cancer, heart disease, stroke, and blood clots compared to postmenopausal women taking a placebo (an inactive pill). However, the increased risks of heart disease were seen only in women several years past the age of menopause, and the risk of breast cancer was rated in the "rare" category, even less than what had been reported in the package insert.

This was *not* a treatment study of younger, midlife menopausal women. It was a study of predominantly older women (ages averaged between 63 and 67) who by and large didn't even have menopausal symptoms anymore. Because this was a preventive study and the bar was set very low for accepting any risk, WHI discontinued the study in this subset of women, saying that the risks were too great to continue—*not* because more women taking hormone therapy were dying than women taking the placebo but because some risks were noted with the treatment arm.

Two years later, the NIH halted another portion of the WHI study, the component investigating PREMARIN, an estrogen-only product.

In this study, participants who were older than 60 had a slightly increased risk of stroke but showed no increase in heart disease and a marked 33 percent decrease in the risk of breast cancer.

By this time, many women who had undergone a hysterectomy had already stopped taking estrogen therapy, spooked by the media reports in 2002. It's ironic that much of their fear centered around the reported increased risks for breast cancer and heart disease, which did not materialize in the estrogen-only trial. Most women don't realize that there's a risk in *not* taking hormone therapy if it's needed. The latest information from the WHI study is that for women who are within 10 years of menopause who have taken HT for 5 or more years there is a 30% reduction in all cause mortality.

So What Are We to Believe About Hormone Therapy?

In my opinion, misunderstanding surrounding the WHI's study design has caused unnecessary panic. This was a prevention—not a treatment—study, and two thirds of the women were over the age of 65, which is 10 to 15 years later than most women would start hormone therapy. The study's purpose was to see whether hormone therapy prevented certain diseases. It was not designed to measure its effectiveness on menopausal symptoms!

Furthermore, the America College of Clinical Endocrinologists announced in 2008 that the benefits of HT in women under age 60 far outweigh the risks. This was based on the reanalysis of data from the WHI in women under age 60, which showed less coronary calcification in women on HT compared to women on no therapy and less overall mortality. It is very concerning that the WHI investigators had this age-stratified data from the beginning but didn't release this important information until years later. The increase in cardiovascular risk that was publicized in 2002 was seen in much older women, over age 70, who were several years from menopause and who were starting "preventive HT" after years of not being exposed to these hormones.

This may be in contrast to older women who have been on HT since the beginning of menopause and done well and not demonstrated any evidence of blood clot. Many of these older women may safely continue on hormone therapy. Furthermore, there was *no* increase in stroke risk in women under age 60.

The bottom-line: *Hormone therapy is still the best treatment for recently menopausal women who are having significant symptoms.*

Women have no reason to fear hormone therapy or to doubt its efficacy as a solution for the uncomfortable and potentially debilitating side effects of menopause. The key is to tailor HT to each woman's individual needs. With so many types of products available, this is easier today than it ever has been before.

What the WHI study showed us is that much older women who do not have any symptoms of menopause should not take hormone therapy solely for "preventive" purposes. In fact, there is not one pill that we encourage all women to take for disease prevention—not aspirin, not vitamin E, and certainly not a single prescription medication. For instance, we advise women at high

Statins and HT: An Interesting Comparison

Like HT, many medications used for prevention, such as statins (cholesterol-lowering medicines), have risks and side effects. However, we don't tell all people with high cholesterol to stop taking their statin just because a small number may have a side effect. Yet this is exactly what happened to millions of women when the proverbial HT rug was pulled out from under them!

Breast cancer rates with statin therapy are comparable to breast cancer rates with HT, and still statin agents are the most commonly prescribed class of medication. Women on HT actually have *reduced* risk of death and cardiovascular mortality if they start HT at the time of menopause—something that cannot be said of statins. What's more, the reduced risk for heart attack in women who use statins has only been shown in women who already have heart disease or who are already at very high risk for heart disease—there isn't yet definitive information on the usefulness of statins as a preventative treatment.

No medicine or substance is perfectly risk-free. That does not mean we don't use these agents. We need perspective, which requires you and your physician to perform an individual risk-benefit assessment. Don't let media hype scare you.

risk for heart disease to take aspirin, and women over the age of 65 are often counseled to consider taking one baby aspirin (81 mg) daily to reduce the risk of stroke by 30 percent. But we do not tell all menopausal women to take aspirin because, for some, the risks of bleeding and other side effects would be greater than the benefits.

The message is that one size does not fit all. All treatments have to be individualized and periodically assessed, and every medicine—prescription as well as nonprescription—carries potential risks as well as potential benefits. We shouldn't throw the baby out with the bath water!

Informing the Debate

You've probably read plenty of contradictory reports by now, leading you to question whether you should start HT or, if you've already started, whether you've put your health in jeopardy just by filling your prescription each month. I hope by reading this book, your anxiety will be quelled.

Let's take a look at some of the most important questions concerning hormone therapy. Here are my conclusions, drawn from careful interpretation of many well-designed scientific studies, as well as years of clinical practice.

What Exactly Is Hormone Therapy?

Hormone therapy supplements the body with estrogen and progestogen (in the form of either synthetic progestins or progesterone). The ovaries are responsible for producing these hormones in women, but during menopause—and especially following complete hysterectomy when the ovaries are removed—we may not produce the amounts needed to regulate certain body functions.

Essentially, by replacing these "missing" hormones with a pill (or in other forms we'll discuss later), the body stays balanced.

Estrogen relieves hot flashes, vaginal dryness, and other symptoms associated with menopause, such as dry, itchy skin. Taken in combination with estrogen, progestin prevents cell overgrowth in the lining of the uterus. This is important in preventing uterine cancer.

Some women prefer estrogen in the form of estradiol, the same estrogen that is produced in the ovary. Other women prefer conjugated estrogens, a mixture of several different estrogens that are either derived from equine urine or synthesized in a lab.

If a woman has had a hysterectomy and is particularly concerned about breast cancer, I recommend PREMARIN (conjugated equine estrogen), as it is the estrogen that has been studied the longest and, in women with hysterectomy, has *not* increased breast cancer. In fact, in the PREMARIN-only arm of the WHI studies, a decreased risk of breast cancer diagnosis was seen. Women who do not want to use an equine source of estrogen may use ENJUVIA (a synthetic form of conjugated estrogens, although not exactly bioequivalent).

Just as many women have preferences regarding the type, dose, and route of estrogen, many women also have strong feelings about progestogens. Once again, one size does not fit all.

Some women prefer to take natural progesterone in the form of PROMETRIUM. (It's mixed in peanut oil, so it's not suitable for women allergic to peanuts.) Other women feel too sleepy on PROMETRIUM, which should always be taken at night. They may prefer other progestins such as norethindrone acetate—found in common birth control pills (such as Loestrin) and in low-dose femhrt and ACTIVELLA (1.0 mg estradiol/0.5 norethindrone acetate and 0.5 mg estradiol/0.1 norethrindone acetate)—or the newer progestin, drospirenone (DRSP), found in ANGELIQ.

Drospirenone is also found in the very popular birth control pills YASMIN and YAZ. Since DRSP is similar to spironolactone, it may provide benefits to skin and hair. It's also a mild diuretic and may lower both blood pressure and cholesterol.

Some women cannot tolerate systemic progestogens and need to use progesterone in the form of a gel such as Prochieve 4%. Other women who have done well on PREMPRO choose to continue it. Now there are lower doses—0.45/1.5 or 0.3/1.5—which have been well studied in the women's HOPE trial, a menopausal treatment study utilizing lower doses of hormone therapy.

Other women who do not want to take a pill or are interested in the transdermal route will use a weekly Climara Pro patch (combining estradiol and levonorgestrel). Women who are concerned about low testosterone may want to use transdermal or vaginal hormones, which do *not* increase SHBG, a sex hormone-binding protein in the liver that lowers testosterone. Conversely, women with too much testosterone, acne, hair thinning, or chin whiskers may want to use an oral estrogen, such as FEMTRACE (estradiol acetate), which raises SHBG and consequently lowers testosterone levels. I favor FEMTRACE over generic estradiol because its level of estrogen is more consistent throughout the day. I also favor brand-name patches such as CLIMARA PRO or VIVELLE-DOT over the larger generic estrogen patches.

Some women who spend lots of time in the water or in humid climates find that the patches don't stick well. Other women want to use transdermal estradiol but don't want to be "marked" by a patch, or they may want to titrate the amount of estrogen they use. These women prefer to use a soybean oil-based lotion (ESTRASORB), an alcohol-based quick-drying gel (like DIVIGEL or ESTROGEL), or a fast-drying estrogen spray (Evamist).

For all the reasons we've discussed so far in this book, many women will continue to turn to HT as a safe, short-term solution for managing severe menopausal symptoms.

Are Older Women Who Take Hormone Therapy at Greater Risk?

Starting HT ten to twenty years after the onset of menopause is generally not advisable, especially if you are taking it solely for non-specific disease prevention or to promote health.

That said, women who are, say, 65 years old, can take hormone therapy to relieve hot flashes, treat genital dryness and sexual dysfunction, and prevent osteoporosis, *if* they started HT at the time of menopause, have done well on the treatment, and want to continue. However, to reduce stroke risk, I favor reducing the dose of estrogen by the time women are between 60 and 65. This is also when we start to talk about preventive aspirin therapy to reduce the risk of stroke and heart attack. (And it's always the right time to talk about smoking cessation, weight reduction, cholesterol control, blood pressure control, and diabetes prevention or treatment.)

As for younger women, the risks found in the WHI do not apply to them. For instance, a 25-year-old woman who finds herself in premature menopause should not identify with the results of research that was done with 65-year-old women.

Are Low Doses of Hormone Therapy Just as Effective as the Previous Standard Doses?

Many times the answer is yes. Low doses of HT are generally effective at treating hot flashes. The hope is that lower doses will assure women that it is okay to start and/or continue hormone therapy, as well as give them more options and dosage ranges.

However, there are no pat answers that apply to all women at all phases of life. Women with severe menopause symptoms may not benefit from low doses as much as they could from a higher dose, which, I remind you, is FDA approved and safe. For example, a woman who suffers from debilitating anxiety attacks coupled with serious hot flashes and very thin bones might fare better with a slightly higher dose of hormones. Furthermore, an "average" dose prescribed for one woman with a fast metabolism may be too low for a woman whose metabolism is slower. Most of the studies that show impressive reductions in osteoporosis and bone breakage have not used the very low doses, so with lower doses, bones need to be monitored. Some women are exceedingly sensitive to hormones, and a low dose may still feel like a high dose to them.

Because each woman's needs are different, you must have a health assessment to determine where you are in the menopause process, whether you are at risk for hormone loss even if you have no menopause symptoms, and at what dose to begin hormone therapy if it will be beneficial for you. (We'll discuss this in more detail in chapter 11.)

Will Hormone Therapy Protect My Heart?

Observations from studies such as the Nurses' Health Study showed a lower incidence of heart disease in women who took hormone therapy. Other studies have found that HT favorably affects lipid levels, meaning that it helps to increase heart-protective HDL cholesterol and decrease dangerous LDL cholesterol.

But in the Heart and Estrogen/Progestin Replacement Study (HERS), postmenopausal women with coronary artery disease did not have a lower rate of cardiac events while taking hormone therapy. And the American Heart Association has issued guidelines stating that hormone therapy should not be used to prevent or treat heart disease, although women who take it for other reasons could continue.

The recent AHA guidelines discourage aspirin use in low-risk women while encouraging its use to reduce the risk of stroke in women in their 60s and beyond. The guidelines also encourage doctors and women to look at lifetime risks for heart disease rather than at immediate risks only.

For instance, a 30-year-old woman who smokes and is overweight is not at immediate risk for heart attack; however, her lifetime risk is very high, and her risk of heart disease should be addressed now. Even a 50-year-old woman who has only one risk factor for heart disease has a substantially increased absolute lifetime risk for both heart disease and a shorter duration of life. Just as HT is not recommended for the prevention of heart disease, SERMs (selective estrogen receptor modulators) such as EVISTA (raloxifene) and the antioxidant vitamins are not recommended for the prevention of heart disease. Women at the very highest risk for heart disease should aim to reduce their LDL cholesterol to under 70, and all women with heart disease should be assessed for depression.

Most recently, WHI findings have discouraged the use of hormone therapy (estrogen-progestin) as a heart-protection drug. However, HT is not damaging to the heart, as some women have been led to believe and when taken at the time of menopause for 5 or more years may actually be beneficial.

This is a lot of information to process and consider. I agree with the WHI guidelines that hormone therapy should not be recommended solely for primary prevention of cardiovascular disease. But even though it can increase the risk of blood clots in a few women predisposed to unusual blood thickening, we shouldn't jump to the conclusion that it causes heart problems.

The bottom line on HT and heart protection is as follows:

- Do not plan on taking hormone therapy to reduce heart attack risk (but it just might in younger women who start out with healthy arteries!)

- Do take it for its therapeutic effects if you need it and are monitored.

- Stay tuned for further research into the potential vascular benefit of estrogen in recently menopausal women with normal arteries, as estrogen may well be cardio-protective for this group of women.

How Will Hormone Therapy Affect Blood Pressure?

Hormone therapy will not have a negative effect on your blood pressure. Actually, many studies have shown that average systolic blood pressure increases less over time in women who take hormone therapy than in women who don't.

Higher doses of oral estrogen, such as in birth control pills or hormonal contraception, can sometimes increase blood pressure.

Does Hormone Therapy Improve Depression?

Estrogen seems to influence the "feel-good" neurotransmitters in the brain (serotonin, dopamine, and norepinephrine). Because the replacement of lost estrogen and, occasionally, progesterone or androgens can improve a woman's self-image and comfort level during menopause, it's reasonable to conclude that hormone therapy does positively influence mood in many but not all women.

But HT might exert benefits beyond helping women regain an "even mood" by eliminating unpleasant symptoms of menopause. When women who had been prescribed estradiol stopped therapy, their hot flashes returned, but their depression did not.

The jury is still out regarding why estrogen has an antidepressant effect in some women. We know only that it's effective in keeping depression at bay while reducing the severe menopausal symptoms that also affect a woman's mood. However, estrogen is not a stand-alone treatment for major depression.

Women who have never had depression, anxiety, or panic attacks but who suddenly develop these symptoms during menopause need to see a women's health specialist who understands the connection in the brain between hormones and neurotransmitters.

Does Hormone Therapy Improve Cognitive Function (Memory and Thought Processes)?

The answer to this controversial question seems to depend on when hormone therapy begins. Some studies show that long-term users of hormone therapy who started using HT at the beginning of menopause show better memory function later in life than women who began to use HT later in their menopause.

Other studies show that starting hormone therapy long after menopause may actually cause some cognitive decline.

Clearly, more research is needed before we can better define the role of hormone therapy in cognitive functioning.

Can Breast Cancer Survivors Use Hormone Therapy?

If you're a breast cancer survivor or receiving treatment for cancer, you must discuss HT with your doctor. Generally, it is not prescribed for women in your situation, since some breast cancers may grow when exposed to estrogen.

There are alternatives, and survivors who have debilitating symptoms of menopause may want to explore low-dose estrogen. The HABITS trial ("Hormonal Replacement Therapy After Breast Cancer—Is It Safe?") showed increased risk of breast cancer recurrence if hormone therapy was used, but other studies have shown no increased risk and perhaps some survival benefit. This may be due to the bias of patient selection for these trials and/or may show different effects, as the trials that used more progestins seem to have worse outcomes.

Certainly, most breast cancer survivors can use ESTRING, a locally applied vaginal estrogen, to restore the integrity of the vagina, as local estrogen therapy does not increase the body's overall exposure to hormones. Many progressive breast cancer specialists allow this use by their patients.

Can We Predict Who Will Benefit From Hormone Therapy and Who Will Be Harmed?

Genetic testing and evolving research will probably allow us to determine in the future who will benefit from long-term HT, as well as those few women who are predisposed to clots and could potentially be harmed.

What we know now is that short-term hormone therapy is safe and effective. It's not a high-risk proposition for those who have discussed this option with their physicians and been found to be suitable candidates. Individualization, monitoring, and re-evaluation are critical. While there is no time limit to hormone therapy, periodic reassessment is needed.

Hormone Therapy: It Works

The WHI study found that 77 percent of women in the study who complained of hot flashes said their flashes diminished while they were on PREMPRO. Bear in mind that women with severe hot flashes were not included in the study, because they would have known right away whether they were taking the drug or a placebo. There are other options for treating hot flashes (see chapter 7), but none is as effective as hormone therapy, which is approved by the FDA for that purpose.

Weighing Risks and Benefits

Again, I stress that hormone therapy is still the best therapy for treating symptoms of menopause. All women should determine their personal risk profile with a knowledgeable physician before starting any prescription treatment.

Having said that, let's look at a summary of the risks and benefits of hormone therapy.

Hormone Therapy Benefits

- Treats hot flashes.
- Prevents osteoporosis.
- Prevents vaginal changes (excessive dryness, thinning tissue).
- May improve skin appearance.
- May reduce the risk for diabetes.
- May reduce the risk for colon cancer (further study is needed).

Hormone Therapy Risks

- Associated with an increased risk of stroke (primarily in older women and with higher doses).

- Can increase risk of gallbladder diseases and need for gallbladder removal.

- Can increase risk of blood clots.

- For women with a uterus (i.e., who have not had a hysterectomy), estrogen used alone can increase risk of uterine cancer. (Estrogen combined with progestin reduces this risk.)

- Has no apparent effect on the risk of ovarian cancer.

Don't forget to put these risks and benefits into context. There is risk in not treating your symptoms, and there is risk in using hormone therapy, just as there is risk in taking or not taking any prescribed therapy.

Is Hormone Therapy Right for Me?

First of all, if you don't feel comfortable taking HT, remember that throughout this book, there are descriptions of alternative treatments in the form of vitamins, foods, and lifestyle changes (exercise, diet, and stress reduction). Some are proven; others are not.

As we've seen, for women with severe menopause symptoms, such alternatives are not enough. Say that you've made the decision to try hormone therapy. How do you know if you are a good candidate?

Your doctor should ask you the following questions:

- Do you have abnormal vaginal bleeding, such as extremely heavy periods or spotting between periods?

- Is there a history of breast cancer in your family?
- Do you have a history of endometrial or uterine cancer?
- Have you ever had venous thrombosis (blood clots in the veins)? This includes thrombosis or blood clots during pregnancy or when taking birth control pills.
- Do you have chronic liver disease?
- Do you smoke?
- Do you have gallbladder disease?

If you answer yes to any of these questions, hormone therapy may not be for you. (In this case, talk with your doctor to learn about other treatment options.) For women with liver disease or increased risks for blood clot or women with gallbladder problems, if HT is going to be used, it would be prudent to use a low dose and go the transdermal route.

But if your answer to every question is no, you are most likely a good candidate for hormone therapy. However, you won't know how well it will work for you until you try it. This is why your physician should start you on a low dose and build gradually, depending on the results.

Am I Better Off With an Alternative?

Some women choose not to start HT for personal reasons. Others should consider alternatives because of existing health conditions. Here are some thoughts on which alternatives might be a good bet for you.

For a Breast Cancer Survivor.

- EFFEXOR XR (venlafaxine) or the new PRISTIQ (desvenlafaxine) for hot flashes (see chapter 11 for details)

- ESTRING or VAGIFEM for vaginal atrophy (see chapter 11 for details)
- Various bone therapy options (see chapter 12 for details)

For a Current Breast Cancer Patient. Women taking TAMOXI-FEN or aromatase inhibitors (AI) are discouraged from any estrogen use, although vaginal estrogen can still be considered.

For a Woman With Predisposed Risk of Breast Cancer. If you do not have hot flashes but are at risk for spine fractures (thin bones) and want to reduce your risk for invasive breast cancer, consider taking daily EVISTA (raloxifene HCI) for five years.

Similar to HT, EVISTA has increased risk for blood clots but does not increase the risk of stroke in older women. However, older women with heart disease who suffer a stroke have an actual increased risk of stroke death if they're taking EVISTA. As with any medication, there are benefits and risks that need to be weighed and factored into your personal situation.

For a Woman With a History of Stroke or Heart Disease. Evaluate and treat cholesterol, blood pressure, and diabetes and stop smoking. Consider using cholesterol-lowering agents and talk to your doctor to see whether you should be on baby aspirin to reduce your risk of heart attack and stroke. Exercise daily. Do not use hormone therapy, EVISTA, and/or antioxidants to prevent heart attack or stroke.

For a Heart Attack Survivor. Even if you've suffered a heart attack, if you're medically stable and your menopause symptoms are severe, HT may still be an option. It's critical to stabilize your status and evaluate all your risks before beginning treatment.

Paradoxically, women who sustain a heart attack while on hormone therapy tend to respond better to treatment than women who have had a heart attack and who are not on HT.

For Someone Experiencing Moderate to Severe Hot Flashes. Hormone therapy is truly the best treatment for hot flashes. Though women try over-the-counter products such as black cohosh, these are generally no more effective than a placebo. In the future, we're likely to have more choices in selecting nonhormonal treatment options to control hot flashes.

For Preventing Osteoporosis. When a woman stops taking hormone therapy, she may experience the rapid bone loss typical of perimenopause and early postmenopause. If the only reason she's taking HT is to prevent osteoporosis, she can use other products to manage rapid bone loss. However, estrogen is the only agent shown to reduce all types of fractures in women who have normal bones and osteopenic bones, as well in women with osteoporosis. (Chapter 12 addresses this further.)

A Final Word on Hormone Therapy and Choice

I am often discouraged by media warnings against hormone therapy. Such reports deal a direct blow to symptomatic women.

Of course, HT should be scrutinized for effectiveness and risks, as should any pharmacological agent. Understanding the risks associated with any therapy is critical before a woman and her physician can make educated decisions together.

The problem occurs when scientific studies are misrepresented in the lay press and blown up into national headlines that do not address the facts underlying a particular study. This happens too often, and the mixed messages confuse women, doing us a great disservice. We feel as if our choices are limited and that our safety is at risk.

If you're suffering from severe menopause symptoms, don't be a martyr. Don't allow yourself to live each day feeling like less of a person because of your discomfort and distress. There are many viable solutions. Hormone therapy is one of them. A solution backed by the FDA, hormone therapy has benefited millions of women and has been shown safe and effective in numerous well-designed studies.

Chapter 11

Customizing Hormone Therapy

Hormone therapy is not a one-size-fits-all solution. Hot flashes may be one woman's most severe menopausal symptom. Her sister may be more concerned about sexual dysfunction. Her best friend may worry about rapid bone loss. Our experience during midlife varies, and menopause symptoms may or may not require treatment with hormone therapy. But if they do, there are many different formulations and a wide variety of types.

Because the women I see in my practice usually have reached their last straw—they are uncomfortable, unhappy, and often desperate—hormone therapy is an option I introduce to them right away.

Many of my patients are already taking some sort type of HT or have filled a prescription for it in the past. But they aren't always taking the right amount or most appropriate type. So sometimes we need to play with the dosage or change the delivery system for better results. Take Miranda for instance.

Miranda

Miranda has a very healthy lifestyle. She exercises daily. She follows an organic vegetarian diet.

She's also always been sensitive and has many allergies. Standard doses of medications are usually too much for her.

When she went through menopause, Miranda was very concerned about taking anything foreign or "synthetic." She didn't want a standard one-size-fits-all treatment but knew she needed something—the hot flashes, vaginal dryness, sleep disturbance, and skin and hair changes made it impossible for her not to seek out some sort of therapy.

Miranda wanted a regimen that would fit in with her lifestyle and a doctor who would support her in using the lowest dose of natural hormone therapy. She had been to various compounding pharmacies but discovered that the standardization and regulation was lacking. Her friend and tennis partner recommended that she see me.

When I saw Miranda, I assured her that one size does not fit all. Since she had had a hysterectomy, we discussed that she would not need to take progesterone and that she only needed to take estrogen, which would relieve her hot flashes; improve her sleep, skin, and hair texture; as well as restore the integrity of the vaginal mucosa. She still had her ovaries in place and was not complaining of any sexual dysfunction or decreased sensation, and she was able to climax although noting that sexual activity was more uncomfortable since entering menopause.

Since she was very sensitive to medications, we decided to use the lowest dose of estrogen. In my office, I showed her a number of different gels. She traveled frequently and did not want to take a large dispenser. Miranda liked the small foil packages of Divigel—a gel that comes in three different strengths. I started her on the very lowest strength, 0.025, and she responded to this within eight weeks; she no longer had significant hot flashes but still had some vaginal dryness. At her follow-up visit, we discussed either increasing the dose of Divigel or adding a local vaginal estrogen cream. Since her bone density was normal, she elected to add just vaginal estrogen and preferred a tablet, Vagifem, inserted twice a week because she was afraid that she would be allergic to the vehicles in the estrogen creams.

Customizing Hormone Therapy

Hormone therapy comes in many forms:

- Pill
- Cream
- Gel
- Tablet
- Vaginal ring
- Spray

One thing that's great about being a midlife woman today is that there are more ways to customize hormone therapy than ever before. Your physician can advise you on which HT delivery method is right for you.

However, do not let swindlers hoodwink you or take advantage by asking you to pay exorbitant fees for extensive testing or tempting you to buy directly from them. Don't believe that their products are safe and totally "risk-free." Nothing is risk-free.

What Kinds of Hormones Does Hormone Therapy Use?

Therapy is *very* personal. Estrogen is great for the vagina, skin, hot flashes, and bones. But for some women—depending on symptoms

Bio-identical HT Versus Bio-similar HT

Bio-identical hormone therapy is catching the attention of women across the country. It simply means using hormones that are identical to human hormones. Bio-similar hormones are the hormones found in hormonal contraceptives and many standardized, well-studied hormone-therapy prescriptions.

and medical history—estrogen is not enough, and other agents are needed. There are several formulations a physician can prescribe:

- Estrogen only
- Estrogen/progestogen (either natural progesterone or a progestin) combination or "cyclical" progesterone added to estrogen
- Estrogen/testosterone combination or compounded testosterone (until the testosterone patch is available)

HT treatments will vary depending on the individual. A woman who has had a complete hysterectomy (removal of the ovaries and uterus) will benefit from estrogen alone, but women who still have a uterus need a progestogen to reduce the risk of uterine cancer. On the other hand, a woman whose primary concern is vaginal atrophy may use local vaginal estrogen therapy only and nothing systemic.

I'd like to take you on a guided tour of various types of HT, so that you can understand some of the options to discuss with your doctor.

Estrogen. This is the hormone therapy prescribed most often. The brand PREMARIN (composed of conjugated equine estrogens) has been available longer than any other and, consequently, has been studied the most extensively.

If a woman is younger than the usual age of menopause and truly needs hormone replacement, her doctor may prescribe ERT (estrogen replacement therapy). If she needs some supplementation to treat problems, her doctor may advise her to take ET (estrogen therapy).

Estrogen comes in various preparations—conjugated estrogens, esterified estrogens, synthetic conjugated estrogen, and estradiol (the most potent human estrogen), as well as ethinyl estradiol, the most common estrogen, which is used in virtually all hormonal contraceptives.

Your physician may recommend a form of treatment that is best for your situation. Also, you may have definite ideas about what treatments you prefer. You can ask your doctor to describe the different options for hormone therapy. This can open the conversation so that you can ask other questions and address all your concerns.

Think about how you'd like to have the hormone delivered. Some women prefer the ease of a pill; others like creams or patches, which bypass the liver and are said to mimic the way the ovary releases estrogen directly into the bloodstream (as opposed to the hormone going through the mouth, stomach, and liver first).

Women who are concerned about their hair and skin might do better taking oral formulations, while women with high triglycerides will not, since oral estrogens may further increase their triglyceride levels.

Women with minor postmenopausal cholesterol problems (such as falling levels of "good" HDL cholesterol and rising levels of "bad" LDL cholesterol) may actually reach better cholesterol ratios with oral formulations rather than transdermal.

As you can see, every regimen has its pros and cons, and every program must be tailored to the needs of the individual.

It's important to remember that if you take oral estrogen, it might reduce your testosterone level. That's a good thing if you're growing a mustache and losing hair on your head, but it's a bad thing if your sex drive is already low.

In general, all brands of estrogens and hormone therapies have similar risks and benefits. Anyone who tells you that their product is completely devoid of potential risks or side effects is lying.

Estrogen/Progestogen (Continuous Combined or Cyclical). Women taking estrogen alone have a two to eight times greater risk of uterine cancer if they take only estrogen and do not balance it with a progestogen. (Remember that *progestogen* is the term that encompasses both progestins—synthetic versions of the hormone progesterone—and progesterone itself.) Because of this risk of uterine cancer, combined estrogen/progestogen therapy is necessary for any woman with a uterus. Progestogens decrease the estrogen-related chance of overgrowth of the lining of the uterus, which can lead to uterine cancer. Studies show that combining estrogen with progestogens completely negates that risk.

If you take combination estrogen/progestogen therapy, you will be on either a "continuous combined" or "cyclic" program.

When progesterone and estrogen are taken together on a daily basis, it is called "continuous combined" therapy. This regimen has the goal of preventing any menstrual-like blood flow, particularly after you have been on it for six months.

With "cyclic," or "sequential," HT, estrogen is taken every day. Progesterone is taken with the estrogen for the first twelve days of the calendar month.

Testosterone: With Estrogen or Compounded. In general, women have more testosterone than estrogen, so calling it a "male sex hormone" is a bit of a misnomer. Men may have ten times more testosterone than women do, but we're certainly not lacking in it—

that is, not until the ovaries are removed and, in some women, after menopause has begun.

For many menopausal women, having extra testosterone may mean having extra side effects, including acne, irritability, and oily skin. But some women with very low testosterone levels see an improvement in sex drive, energy, muscle mass, and bone with testosterone. And one in six women may need testosterone after undergoing a hysterectomy. (See chapter 9.)

Currently, the only way to take testosterone for menopause is in a formulation that combines it with estrogen. There are two products—ESTRATEST HS and SYNTEST HS—that combine oral esterified estrogen with methyltestosterone (a synthetic form of oral testosterone).

Although there is no FDA-approved way to give testosterone transdermally to women, a female testosterone patch, called INTRINSA, looks promising. It has been approved in Europe already, and it should be available to women in North America soon.

I think the testosterone patch should have been approved in the United States already. Unfortunately, it came up for FDA approval right after the controversy about the safety of the arthritis drug VIOXX. To my way of thinking, the FDA advisory committee was being overly conservative and paternalistic.

The all-male panel was not particularly impressed by the fact that INTRINSA's formulation helped improve women's sexual activity by "only one extra episode of sexual activity per month," even though for many women it's the quality, not the quantity of sexual encounters that's important. Women in the study reported that their sexual satisfaction significantly improved compared to baseline. In fact, many participants wanted to stay on the patch after the study ended. I think women—with the help of a knowledgeable physician, of course—should have the option of deciding what is best for them. Recently, INTRINSA has been studied in postmenopausal women not on estrogen and has shown improvement in sexual function.

Meanwhile, the topical testosterone preparations currently available are formulated for men, not for women, who can use only one-tenth of the dosage. This is why many doctors use compounding pharmacies when women require testosterone. Most of us would rather be able to prescribe an agent like the INTRINSA patch—something that would allow us to know exactly how much hormone a woman is being exposed to. Our current situation involves too much guesswork and, ironically, may put women at greater risk than if the FDA had approved the patch for women.

Types of Delivery Systems

Numerous FDA-approved options provide women with more HT choices. There are several main formulations.

Most hormone therapies are available in pill form. They come in ultra-low, low-, medium-, intermediate-, higher-, and highest-dose formulas. Generally, women who have undergone hysterectomies, have experienced chemotherapy-induced menopause, or are very young may need higher doses to control hot flashes and other menopause concerns.

For most women, the physician will start you on a low dose and monitor you for at least three to eight weeks before increasing it. Other physicians may start with a higher dose to control symptoms faster and then reduce the dosage.

Estrogen-only Pills

- **PREMARIN.** A complex blend of multiple conjugated equine estrogens (CEE); taken daily (doses: 0.3, 0.45, 0.625, 0.9, 1.25, 2.5 mg).

- **ENJUVIA.** Synthetic conjugated estrogens; similar to PREMARIN but not bioequivalent; taken daily (doses: 0.3, 0.45, 0.625, 1.25 mg).

- **FEMTRACE.** Generic name: estradiol acetate (E2). Lastwenty-four hours (doses: 0.45, 0.9, 1.8 mg), as opposed to the generic estradiol formulation, which should be taken twice a day.

- **MENEST.** Esterified estrogen; taken daily (doses: 0.3, 0.625, 1.25, 2.5 mg).

- **Ethinyl estradiol (EE).** This higher-dose synthetic is generally not used for menopausal purposes except in very low doses found in femhrt 5 mcg and femhrt low-dose 2.5 mcg. (EE is used in most birth control pills in doses of 20, 25, 30, 35, 50 mcg.)

Estrogen/Progestin

This is used by women with a uterus who want the convenience of one pill or one patch without cycling or withdrawal bleeding:

- **PREMPRO.** Medroxyprogesterone acetate; daily pill (dose: 0.625 mg/2.5 mg).

- **PREMPRO low-dose versions.** Daily pill (doses: 0.45 mg/ 1.5 mg and 0.3 mg/1.5 mg).

- **ACTIVELLA.** Daily pill (dose: 1.0 mg/0.5 mg).

- **ACTIVELLA low-dose version.** Daily pill (dose 0.5 mg/ 0.1 mg).

- **FEMHRT.** Daily pill (dose: 5 mcg/1.0 mg).

- **FEMHRT low-dose version.** Daily pill (dose: 2.5 mcg/1.0 mg).

- **ANGELIQ.** Daily pill (dose: 1 mg estradiol/0.5 mg DRSP).

- **CLIMARA Pro.** Weekly patch. (dose: 0.045 mg/0.015 mg).

- **COMBIPATCH.** Patch, changed twice a week. (dose: 0.05 mg/ 0.14 mg or 0.05 mg/0.25 mg).

Estrogen/Testosterone

This can be used by women who have had hysterectomies or by women who still have their uteruses in combination with a progestogen.

- **ESTRATEST HS.** Oral pill of esterified estrogens and methyltestosterone.
- **SYNTEST HS.** Oral pill of esterified estrogens and methyltestosterone.

Progesterone

- **PROMETRIUM (natural micronized progesterone).** Pill, taken orally at night (dose: 200 mg or 100 mg). This can be taken either cyclically or nightly in combination with any type of estrogen.
- **PROCHIEVE 4% (progesterone gel).** Vaginal gel used every other night for the first twelve days of the calendar month.

Progestins

- **PROVERA (MPA).** This is taken orally, usually in combination form. (It was the progestin used in the WHI study.)
- **Micronor norethindrone acetate (NA).** This is taken orally. It is commonly found in birth control pills, as well as some HT pills.
- **MIRENA (levonorgestrel).** This intrauterine system (IUS) is used for contraception, but can be used off-label to reduce

menstrual bleeding or to protect locally the lining of the uterus in women who are taking systemic estrogen.

- **Cyclical progestogens added to estrogen.**

- **PREMPHASE.** Daily pill (0.625 CEE/cycled 5 mg of MPA).

- **PREFEST.** Daily pill (estradiol with cyclical norgestimate).

- **Any estrogen estradiol.** Oral (e.g., Femtrace), patch (e.g., Climara), or topical individualized bioidentical estrogen (e.g., Divigel, Evamist, or Estrasorb) can be used daily, and then any progestogen (usually PROMETRIUM) can be added for twelve days a month.

Women with a uterus who request "bio-identical" HT and want only the hormones their bodies have made or been "naturally" exposed to are frequently happy with one of these regimens.

Transdermal Estrogen

Lotion/Gel. A soy-based emulsion containing bio-identical estrogen/estradiol is applied to legs or skin on a daily basis to treat hot flashes and night sweats. The lotion has a soybean oil base. Some women like the moisturization; others do not like the oily feel or smell.

- **DIVIGEL.** An estradiol gel that comes in three strengths (0.1, 0.05, 0.025) and is the most concentrated and hence smallest amount of gel. Comes in a small foil package that provides a convenient transdermal option and allows you and your physician to find the optimal dose.

- **ESTRASORB.** This estradiol lotion comes in two foil packets and allows the woman flexibility in controlling the amount she uses.

- **ESTROGEL.** This alcohol-based gel is delivered by metered squirts and applied to skin on the arms daily. (The European dose is two squirts a day; the one squirt a day of the American regimen is a very low dose.)

- **EVAMIST.** This is the newest transdermal estrogen. It is a spray that is approved for one to three sprays onto the arm daily. Each dispenser contains 60 sprays and needs to be first primed with three squirts. Evamist has the convenience of fast application without getting any estrogen on the hand. Interestingly the levels of estrogen, while low, appear to peak around 3 AM, which may help with sleep and night sweats reduction.

- **ELESTRIN.** Another topical estrogen gel.

- **Vaginal cream.** Creams are generally used only to treat vaginal symptoms, including dryness, itching, and burning in and around the vagina. There are several brands available, including ESTRACE vaginal cream (estradiol) and PREMARIN vaginal cream (CEE).

Vaginal Ring

- **ESTRING.** This very low-dose vaginal ring is a small, circular piece of silastic plastic containing a tiny amount of estradiol. The comfortable ring is easily inserted like a diaphragm into the vagina. It releases steady doses of estrogen for three months at a time. Rings can treat vaginal dryness and hot flashes and, in higher doses, bone effects. It's frequently used in women who otherwise cannot take or tolerate estrogen, such as women with a history of breast cancer or blood clots.

- **FEMRING.** This is available in two doses (0.05 and 0.10) for both vaginal and systemic treatment, renewed every three months. It's usually used in women who've had a hysterectomy and want the local and systemic benefits of estrogen.

What Is the Difference Between Bio-identical Hormones and Conjugated Estrogens?

Bio-identical hormones are identical in molecular structure to the hormones created in women's bodies. They're not found in this form in nature but are made or synthesized from plant chemicals.

Conjugated estrogens are a mixture of several different estrogens that are either derived from equine urine or synthesized in a lab.

Vaginal Tablet. Tablets are inserted into the vagina with an applicator and may be less messy than vaginal creams. Tablets generally relieve vaginal symptoms and, like ESTRING, have been shown to reduce the risk of recurrent bladder infections.

- **VAGIFEM.** This is applied to the lower third of the vagina twice a week.

Estrogen Patches. Patches treat hot flashes and other menopause symptoms. They range in size from smaller than a dime to the size of a half-dollar. They're applied to the abdomen or lower back area and will usually stay on while you're showering or swimming. Some last one week; others must be changed twice a week.

Examples of some estrogen-only patches include the following:

- **CLIMARA Pro.** This estradiol patch is changed weekly (doses: 0.025, 0.0375, 0.050, 0.060, 0.075, 0.100).

- **VIVELLE-DOT.** This estradiol patch is changed twice a week (doses: 0.0375, 0.050, 0.075, 0.100). The 0.025 dose of Vivelle-Dot is only for bone health and not hot flash control. Regardless of dose size, all women who are taking Vivelle-Dot and still have a uterus must also use progestogen monthly.

- **MENOSTAR.** Menostar is the lowest-dose estrogen patch available (dose: 0.014 mg). The dose is so low that it is not specifically approved for the treatment of hot flashes. Rather, it has been studied in women ages 60 to 80 who no longer have hot flashes but have bone thinning/osteopenia and want to use this weekly patch for osteoporosis prevention. The dose is low enough that a woman with a uterus needs to use a progestogen only once or twice a year (rather than monthly, as is the case with the other strengths of estrogen).

Which Delivery System Is Best?

I like to show women in my practice all the different types of hormones so that they can chose the one that is most convenient and that best fits with their lifestyle.

I find women who live in humid environments or who perspire a lot do not like patches. Women who travel like the tiny foil applicators, like DIVIGEL, and women who want a fast drying quick method without the need to wash estrogen gel off their hands prefer EVAMIST spray. Other women prefer to take oral estrogen. I prefer oral PREMARIN (conjugated estrogens) or FEMTRACE (estradiol) because they last at least 24 hours.

A Word About Generics

I do not like patients to use generic estradiol, as the half-life is quick and it needs to be dosed orally at least twice a day. Furthermore, I like my patients to avoid any generic hormones as generics only have to be 80 percent to 125 percent equivalent to brand name—

Questions to Ask Your Doctor

- Why should I take hormone therapy?
- Which HT delivery method is right for me?
- Do I need both estrogen and progesterone?
- What is the lowest available dose of hormone therapy?
- How long should I take it?
- What are possible side effects?
- What are the risks?

that simply is too wide a range for a potent substance like a hormone. Also, the strengths between generic batches can vary, so every month can feel like a hormonal roller coaster with varying levels. The same is true for generic thyroid hormone and bone medications—I usually only prescribe the brand name because that is what I personally would want for myself or a family member to take.

Birth Control for Perimenopausal Women

The birth control pill is an effective way to reduce menopausal symptoms in women who haven't completely stopped having periods. At this time, a woman may still need pregnancy protection, so the pill is a logical and safe option for healthy women who do not smoke or have a history of medical problems. In addition to providing contraception, the pill will curb the hot flashes, night sweats, and irritability associated with menopause.

Birth control pills have also been shown to reduce bone loss and the risk of ovarian cancer, and they do not increase the risk of breast cancer. Women taking the pill or any form of hormonal contraceptives (HC) tend to have lighter and less painful periods.

Women who are nonsmokers and in general good health can take birth control until they are 55 years old. After a woman starts menopause, I recommend that she stop taking birth control. Any form of any hormone, including HT and HC, can increase the risk of blood clots. In general, this is the most serious risk.

Low-dose birth control pills can deliver up to five times as much estrogen as hormone therapy. So when a woman is on the pill, she gets enough estrogen to prevent those ovaries from releasing an egg. But some women experience menopause symptoms during the week they take the "inactive" pills. When the active pills are resumed the following week, the symptoms disappear.

If you're in this situation, you have a choice. You don't have to have a period, and you don't have to take the "inactive" pills if you have menopausal symptoms. In fact, the initial design of an active pill taken for twenty-one days followed by seven days of "inactive" pills is rapidly becoming obsolete. Seven days is a long time to go without hormones, especially when symptoms might include menstrual migraines, painful periods, mood changes, and/or peri-menopausal breakthrough symptoms.

You might want to consider one of the new pill options that come under the 24/4 regimen. This means your pill pack comes with twenty-four active hormone pills and only four inactive/dummy pills. Examples of newer products include the following:

- **LOESTRIN 24 Fe.** (dose: 20 mcg EE and 1 mg NA)
- **YAZ.** (dose: 20 mcg EE and 3mg DRSP) A 24/4 day pill, YAZ is the only pill that is FDA-approved to treat severe PMS. It is also indicated to treat acne. It has a favorable progestogen, drospirenone (DRSP), which contains a spiro-nolactone analogue and seems particularly beneficial for skin and hair concerns. Also, it is not associated with bloating, which can occur with some progestins.

  If a woman has done well on YASMIN or YAZ and is now in menopause, I favor using ANGELIQ for HT.

Similarly, if she has done well on Loestrin, then I would consider transitioning her to femhrt, which has the same constituents but at a lower dose.

- **SEASONALE.** This is the first long-cycle pill to contain twelve weeks of active pills and one week of inactive pills, leading to one menstrual cycle once a season.

- **SEASONIQUE.** This works the same as SEASONALE, but the last week's dose contains a small amount of ethinyl estradiol to reduce the incidence of hormone withdrawal symptoms.

- **LYBREL.** This was the first 365-day pill available, meaning that an active pill is taken daily, with no breaks and no periods. Actually, any hormonal contraceptive can be used in a continuous daily fashion to avoid any drops in hormone levels. For women with menstrual migraines, hormone sensitivities, hot flashes, or sleep disturbance with placebo use, a continuous regimen is very beneficial.

If You're on the Pill, How Can You Tell When You Start Menopause?

You can test yourself by stopping the pill to see whether you still get your period. If you're sexually active, there's a chance you can still get pregnant, so you should use a backup form of contraception at this time. You must be off hormonal contraception for several months before a physician can correctly interpret the lab tests and determine your hormone status.

Hormone Therapy and Quality of Life

Many women who take hormone therapy say they just feel better taking it than they do without it. They have fewer problems with their skin, vaginal atrophy, sexuality, sleep, mood, cognitive function, and hot flashes. You can't measure these considerations as easily as you can measure body weight or blood pressure or cholesterol levels. Nonetheless, they hold particular importance for many women. And because there is no one therapy that addresses all these concerns, many women find that HT remains their best bet.

If you've been taking hormone therapy for four years, your physician may wish to taper your HT dosage to test the waters and find out whether you can get by with less or no hormone therapy and still maintain optimum health and a high quality of life.

Here are some reasons that your physician may recommend tapering hormone therapy:

- You no longer have menopausal symptoms.
- You're concerned about prolonged use of an HT that contains progestins, which have been linked to a slightly higher risk of breast cancer, and/or you're approaching age 60 and are concerned about an increased risk of stroke, which has been noted in older women on both estrogen and estrogen/progestogen therapy.
- You're not deriving any benefit from HT.
- You're experiencing side effects such as breast tenderness, bleeding, or bloating.

When women stop taking hormone therapy abruptly, they may experience these side effects:

- Insomnia, night sweats
- Irritability
- Bone loss
- Vaginal thinning

HT Time Frames

Some women never need HT, some women need HT for a limited time, and many women need HT indefinitely. Women who have stopped systemic HT or who have never used any HT may very well need local vaginal estrogen therapy.

There's no time limit to the use of HT, but there's a need to re-evaluate your need for it periodically, as with any therapy. For women who start HT around the time of menopause and continue it for five or more years, they actually tend to have less heart disease, less coronary calcifications, and a lower death rate! So I am not in any hurry to tell a woman arbitrarily she has to stop hormones. I ask her to listen to her body and periodically get re-evaluated. As a woman ages, metabolism changes, so a lower dose of hormones may be as effective as a higher dose was when she was younger.

Slowly tapering off HT does not necessarily make it less likely that a woman will suffer from symptoms. Interestingly, there is a lack of research in this area, so I take the lead from the woman herself, asking her what she'd like to do.

However, if you're no longer on HT or never took HT, you have to pay particular attention to the status of your bones and vagina because these are the areas of the body particularly sensitive to loss of estrogen.

Again, remember that there is no time limit on the use of HT. The goal is to have neither too few nor too many hormones but just the right amount. Determining your optimal hormone balance means listening to your body and seeing an experienced physician if problems arise.

For example, trying to determine the right hormone balance for a woman is much more complicated than determining whether her thyroid hormone is too high or too low. While many women require lifelong thyroid hormone therapy, others never need thyroid hormone, just as there are women who never need HT or need it only for a relatively short time. That said, at least half of all women lose bone after menopause, and without estrogen, most women will experience some thinning and atrophy of the reproductive and urinary system systems.

Here's another example. Millions of women have benefited from taking the pill, a synthetic combination of estrogen and progestin. In human history, no other agent has been studied so much, and by allowing women some reliable control over reproduction for the first time in history, it's the one pharmaceutical that has revolutionized women's lives. Nonetheless, many women have never used the pill or any form of hormonal contraception, preferring to avoid not only synthetic hormones but hormone therapy of any sort. Others, who never needed the pill or perhaps were unable to take it, still may be interested in HT. So again, one size, one prescription does not fit all!

Younger women have many choices when it comes to controlling their bodies' reproductive and menstrual cycles. Midlife women should have just as many ways to maximize their health and vitality.

Hormone therapy should be one of their options.

Chapter 12

Boosting Bone Health

Midlife is a critical turning point for a woman's bone health. There's a direct relationship between menopause and the development of the bone-thinning disorder osteoporosis. In the five to seven years following menopause, a woman can lose up to 20 to 30 percent of her bone mass. And when a woman experiences early menopause, she is especially at risk for rapid bone loss.

This makes midlife a prime time to prevent and treat low bone density so that we can stay strong in later years. And yet, so many women don't realize or aren't advised by their doctors to begin testing for bone loss early. Elisa's experience is far too common.

Elisa

I'm 52 years old and have officially entered menopause, so I felt it would be a good idea to see a physician who specializes in women's health. But when my new doctor suggested that I get a bone mineral density (BMD) test, I was skeptical. My former doctor always told me that a BMD test before age 65 was a waste. He said, "No risk factors, no reason to get the test."

My new doctor explained that this was very old-fashioned thinking. She said that even without risk factors, every woman should have a BMD test within two years of menopause. She told me that just being female is a risk factor for loss in bone density because of the metabolic changes and estrogen deficiency we experience after menopause.

I got the test my new physician ordered, and the results surprised me—I was diagnosed with osteopenia. The doctor explained that this didn't necessarily mean I had a disease. It meant I have lower bone density than some other women my age. It also meant that I could be losing bone and that I'm at higher risk than an average woman for bone breakage, especially as I get older.

If the new doc hadn't tested my BMD, I'd have continued to assume that my bones were strong. You can't see or feel a loss in bone density.

As it turns out, my past doctor's claim that I didn't display risks was dead wrong. The brush-off he gave me about not needing a BMD at my age is scary. I wonder how many other women simply trust their doctor's orders without getting a second opinion?

What Is Osteopenia?

Osteopenia is a condition characterized by decreased calcification (deposits of calcium salts, which are needed to form bone), decreased density, or reduced bone mass. It may warrant pharmacological treatment. A diagnosis of osteopenia means that you have less bone mass than the average woman.

Having less bone mass than average is not necessarily a problem—just as being shorter than the average woman isn't usually a problem. However, once you establish your baseline bone density, if you start losing bone rapidly, it's a problem and needs to be addressed. The less dense your bones are, the more likely you are to break one.

What Exactly Is Osteoporosis?

Osteoporosis is the loss of normal bone density, mass, and strength, leading to increased porosity and vulnerability to fracture. Type 1 osteoporosis is related to menopause and is almost always preventable. Type 2 osteoporosis is related to aging and affects older men and women over age 65, but it is still modifiable and manageable. Our focus here is on Type 1.

Osteoporosis is *not* a normal part of aging. It can be prevented and treated, though there is no cure. The key is to identify rapid loss in bone density during postmenopausal years so that you can take action to slow the process and, in some cases, stop it and even rebuild bone. This is very important as it will protect you from debilitating bone fractures.

A number of approved options exist to prevent and manage osteoporosis, one of which is hormone therapy. If you recently started menopause, knowing your bone status may affect your decision about whether to use HT or other treatments for your menopausal bone loss.

Who Gets Osteoporosis?

Eighty percent of people with osteoporosis are women. But osteoporosis is mistakenly thought of as a disease only of older white women. Or as a problem of skinny women. Neither of these assumptions is true.

In fact, in the United States, osteoporosis and low bone mass affect 44 million women and men age 50 and older, according to the National Osteoporosis Foundation. That's 55 percent of people in that age group.

At least one in two white women over age 50 will have an osteoporosis-related fracture in her lifetime. Women of color may be less likely to develop osteoporosis, but they still are at risk. Ten percent of African American women over age 50 have osteoporosis; an additional 30 percent have low bone density, putting them at risk for osteoporosis. And women of color who sustain a hip fracture are more likely to die from it than white women. Unfortunately, some physicians don't even realize that many of their women patients of color are at risk for osteoporosis, so you may need to speak up for yourself . . . or switch doctors!

• • • **Fast Fact** • • •

1.5 million fractures per year are due to osteoporosis.

• • •

If I Exercise and Take Calcium Supplements, Can I Avoid Osteoporosis?

Some people think that if they simply exercise and take calcium supplements, they will be protected from osteoporosis. Although exercise, calcium, and vitamin D are a good start, they're not the only ways you should protect yourself from bone loss. A number of factors affect a woman's predisposition for osteoporosis, including age and hormonal status. You can exercise and drink milk until the cows come home but still lose bone.

You and your doctor should also take into account your

- diet and exercise.
- family history.
- weight.
- smoking.
- history of eating disorders.
- history of kidney stones; some women excrete too much calcium in their urine.

- history of wheat/gluten intolerance (celiac disease), which reduces the body's ability to absorb enough vitamin D and iron.

You can get calcium from foods, but chances are slim that you're meeting all your calcium needs through your diet and even slimmer you are ingesting enough vitamin D. (We'll talk more about supplements in a moment.)

Bone Basics

You may associate bones with a hard and lifeless skeleton. In fact, bone is a complex living tissue. The bones' innermost layer, the marrow, makes blood cells, which keep us alive. Bones also provide structural support for muscles, protect our vital organs, and store calcium.

Bones are in a continuous cycle of repeated breakdown and buildup known as "remodeling." During the phase of the cycle called "resorption," bones release calcium into the blood, which

When Is a Broken Bone Not a Broken Bone?

If you or your child has had a broken bone that healed well, all this talk about bone fractures may strike you as odd. Bones break, are set, and heal, right? Not necessarily. Not when we're older.

Statistics show that almost 40 percent of elderly people who have a hip fracture die within the following year. They may die from complications from the fracture or its treatment or from having been immobilized during recovery. Those who survive run the risk of losing their independence.

results in bone breakdown. In the "formation" phase, new bone is built to replace the old. This ongoing cycle of replacing old bones with new ones gives the body the calcium it needs while keeping the skeleton strong.

When formation exceeds resorption, the bone mass increases. But if resorption is faster than formation, there's a reduction in bone mass. When the bone mass is continually reduced, it leads to osteoporosis.

How Is Bone Mass Built Up?

From infancy up until age 30, human beings build more bone than they lose. After 30, we maintain our bone density, and later in life we try to prevent its loss.

Think of it this way. Each of us maintains a lifelong "bone bank," and we constantly make deposits and withdrawals depending on lifestyle choices, such as getting enough calcium and exercising regularly. Some of us with family histories of osteoporosis who are naturally thin or small-framed, or who suffer fractures after the age of 40, automatically start with a lower "balance" in that bank. We have to work harder to keep it full.

The catch: By age 30, when most of us have acquired most of our skeletal mass, we can't make any more deposits.

Following menopause, the ovaries usually stop producing enough bone-protecting hormones, which can increase the rate of "withdrawals" from the bone bank. Over time, without treatment, the increased withdrawals take their toll. Osteoporosis increases the risk of fracture and, in more serious cases, can reduce mobility.

The good news is that you can increase bone mass during midlife and prevent loss during menopause with hormone therapy and/or other pharmacological options designed for women who are at high risk or who've had actual bone loss.

What Are the Risk Factors for Osteoporosis?

You can't always tell whether someone has osteoporosis, especially when it's in the early stages and in active midlife women who don't "look the part." Also, osteoporosis doesn't usually cause symptoms until you break a bone.

However, certain women are more likely to develop osteoporosis and fractures. In fact, simply by being a woman, your risk for low bone mass automatically increases. Such metabolic changes as menopause-related hormone loss also increase your risk. And if you've been ignoring your daily calcium and vitamin D intake, you're not doing your part to prevent your bones from weakening.

Early awareness, regular weight-bearing exercises such as walking or lifting small weights, and making sure that you take enough calcium and vitamin D are key. Talk to your doctor to make sure you are doing enough.

Here are the risk factors:

- Estrogen deficiency after menopause.
- Having a thin or small frame.
- A family history of osteoporosis; history of fracture in a close relative.
- A personal history of fracture (after age 40).
- A history of amenorrhea (absence of menstrual periods for several months at a time).
- A history of disordered eating.
- A low lifetime intake of calcium and vitamin D.
- Smoking cigarettes.
- Excessive alcohol use.
- An inactive lifestyle.
- Advanced age.

Red Flag

Osteoporosis is called the "silent disease" because it progresses slowly, often without symptoms until a fracture occurs. At this point, a person has already suffered the consequences of low bone density.

Also, many women assume that height loss is a normal part of aging, but it may be due to collapse in spinal bones weakened by osteoporosis. That's why it's so important to measure your height yearly. If your height changes by more than an inch, report it to your physician.

- The presence of certain chronic medical conditions (including rheumatoid arthritis, celiac disease, and anorexia nervosa).

- Use of certain medications, including steroids, glucocorticoids, and aromatase inhibitors such as AROMASIN (exemestane), FEMARA (letrozole), and ARIMIDEX (anastrozole), as well as LUPRON or other medications that stop monthly periods. (Medications that stop periods wipe out all estrogen and put women at risk for osteoporosis. This is in contrast to hormonal contraceptives taken continuously that do not stimulate a "withdrawal" period but still give daily, continuous estrogen and actually protect the bones.

- The presence of a malabsorption condition, such as celiac or gluten enteropathy (wheat-protein intolerance).

Assessing Bone Health: The BMD Test

As you enter menopause, it is a good time to assess how strong your bones are. Your physician will determine whether you need a bone mineral density test based on your clinical history and risk factors.

A BMD test will do the following:

- Measure the mineral density in your bones. The amount of certain minerals, such as calcium, in your bones is an indicator of their health and strength.
- Assess your risk for fracture.
- Determine your rate of bone loss and/or monitor the effects of treatment if the test is conducted at intervals of two or more years.

Generally, the lower your bone mineral density, the higher your risk of fracture and osteoporosis.

What Happens During a BMD Test?

BMD X-ray tests are quick and painless, and there are various methods of measuring bone density. Depending on your needs, your physician may order a test using a peripheral X-ray machine that measures density in the finger, wrist, kneecap, shinbone, and heel. Central X-ray machines gather bone density measurements from the hip, spine, and total body, which is the gold standard of measurement.

During a BMD test, you lie flat on your back on a padded table. An X-ray machine projects beams onto the targeted bone areas. The amount of the beam that is blocked by bone indicates density, enabling a physician to compare results with bone density standards. This is like getting a quick snapshot of your bone health.

Bone Density and the Decision for Hormone Therapy

The estrogen in hormone therapy can improve or stabilize women's bone health. So knowing their bone status and their rate of bone loss helps many recently postmenopausal women decide whether they want to begin to use HT.

The DXA: Measuring Bone Mineral Density

There are different types of machines to measure bone density. Some are portable, but these are not considered as reliable as larger models.

A common reliable bone test is DXA (dual energy X-ray absorptiometry), which measures the thickness of bone at the spine, hip, or total body. The bone thickness (bone mineral density) is measured using two levels of X-ray energy.

A woman with severe menopausal symptoms (vaginal atrophy, hot flashes, and skin changes) may be able to choose a therapy for her symptoms that also prevents rapid bone loss. So her physician might order a BMD test to determine her bone status and factor the result into recommendations concerning hormone therapy.

When Should I Get a BMD Test?

I recommend BMD testing within two years of menopause—earlier for patients with a family history of osteoporosis, low vitamin D levels, or long-term steroid medication use and for women who have unexplained bone fractures, skipped menses, or taken treatments that lower their hormone levels.

Scoring Your Test: From T to Z

The result of a BMD is either a T-score or a Z-score.

T-scores. A T-score compares your bone density to an ideal number (that of a healthy 30-year-old female). If your bone density is the same as the ideal, your score is 0. If your bone is more or less dense than the ideal, it's measured in units called standard deviations. If your score is within one standard deviation of the ideal (i.e., from −1 to +1), you have normal bone density. Numbers falling below −1 indicate that the bone is thinning. The lower the T-score, the higher the risk of a fracture.

The following are criteria set by the World Health Organization. They list four diagnostic categories based on the T-score:

- Normal: Above +1.0 to −1.0

- Osteopenia: −1.1 to −2.4

- Osteoporosis: Greater than or equal to −2.5

- Severe or established osteoporosis: A T-score of less than or equal to −2.5 with a known fracture

However, the National Osteoporosis Risk Assessment trial revealed that postmenopausal women with peripheral T-scores of −1.7 or less were also at risk for fracture.

This is why factors such as age, body weight, and history combined with T-scores can further quantify fracture risk and treatment needs and why you should always consult a knowledgeable physician about your bone health rather than trusting a single number.

Z-scores. The Z-score compares your bone density to that of someone of your own age and ethnic group. It can be used in premenopausal women (who usually don't need a bone density test). A Z-score can also be used to compare postmenopausal women to their own peers, as well as to the T-score standard for normal young adults.

If a woman has a low Z-score, meaning that not only is she low compared to the average 30-year-old woman but is really low compared to a woman of her own age and ethnicity, it should be taken as a warning that her bone thinning may be due to something other than her age and postmenopausal status.

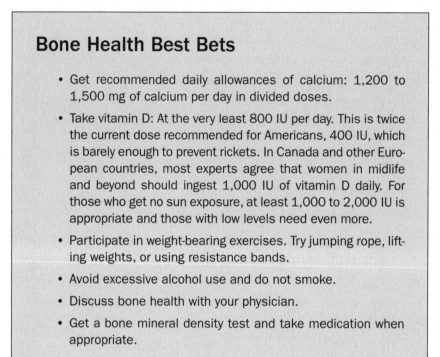

Bone Health Best Bets

- Get recommended daily allowances of calcium: 1,200 to 1,500 mg of calcium per day in divided doses.
- Take vitamin D: At the very least 800 IU per day. This is twice the current dose recommended for Americans, 400 IU, which is barely enough to prevent rickets. In Canada and other European countries, most experts agree that women in midlife and beyond should ingest 1,000 IU of vitamin D daily. For those who get no sun exposure, at least 1,000 to 2,000 IU is appropriate and those with low levels need even more.
- Participate in weight-bearing exercises. Try jumping rope, lifting weights, or using resistance bands.
- Avoid excessive alcohol use and do not smoke.
- Discuss bone health with your physician.
- Get a bone mineral density test and take medication when appropriate.

A Z-score of −1.5 to −2.0 below the mean age indicates a possible need to evaluate for secondary causes of bone loss. These causes could include the following:

- Vitamin D deficiency
- Low estrogen states
- Hyperparathyroidism
- Overactive thyroid
- Elevated cortisol levels
- Malabsorption of needed nutrients
- Hormone imbalance
- Multiple myeloma

Vitamin D

Adults need at least 1,000 to 2,000 IUs of Vitamin D daily. Vitamin D is fat soluble and can be taken all at once. Overweight patients with low vitamin D levels take longer to normalize as vitamin D is fat soluble. Up to 10,000 IU of vitamin D3 could be taken daily for several months prior to developing elevated levels. When patients are low in vitamin D, prescription ergocalciferol (D2) is prescribed in 50,000 IU twice a week for a few months with a recheck of the 25-OH vitamin D level.

Prescription vitamin D is used to "fill up the tank" to normal. If you fill up the tank but neglect to gas up regularly with daily vitamin D3, you will just run on empty again.

- Use of certain medications
- Excessive loss of calcium through the urine

When Should I Seek Treatment?

As I noted previously, I recommend BMD testing within two years of menopause and earlier for patients with a family history of osteoporosis, low vitamin D levels, and/or long-term steroid use (7.5 mg of prednisone or more for three or more months). The decision to treat a postmenopausal woman for osteoporosis or low bone density/osteopenia should be based on a combination of T-scores and the clinical risk factors already noted. Postmenopausal women who show marked or significant decreases in bone density (in comparison to previous years' BMD test results) are also candidates for treatment.

A combination of good health and exercise, supplementation with calcium and vitamin D, and possibly a regimen of either hormone therapy or a prescribed bone therapy can treat osteopenia, prevent osteoporosis, and reduce your risk of bone breakage and height loss (dowager's hump).

Bone Therapies

Depending on the severity of bone loss, a woman may be able to improve her bone density through lifestyle changes alone, such as increasing her calcium and vitamin D intake, and doing weight-bearing exercise. But this is not enough for many women.

There are FDA-approved medications that prevent or slow down loss of bone density. And for menopausal women who are at high risk of developing osteoporosis (or who already are rapidly losing bone mass), hormone therapy in a pill or patch form is an option that I highly recommend. If you can't take hormone therapy or don't want to, there are other options. If bone density is your only postmenopausal concern, then you should consider other agents besides HT.

Bisphosphonates

Bisphosphonates are antiresorptive treatments; they slow or stop the dissolving of bone tissue in the normal bone cycle (described earlier) without slowing down formation of new bone tissue. This means that formation occurs faster than resorption, so bone density may increase over time—at the very least, a woman will not lose bone faster than she can replace it. These treatments include the following:

- **ACTONEL (risedronate).** Dose: 35 mg weekly (or 5 mg daily); recently, this has become available in once monthly 150 mg doses. ACTONEL reduces the risk of all types of fractures (vertebral/spine and nonvertebral fractures, including hip, pelvis, wrist, and humerus) and is the only bisphosphonate FDA approved to prevent glucocoricoid (steroid) induced osteoporosis. After taking ACTONEL with plain tap water, you must wait at least 30 minutes prior to eating or drinking other beverages. ACTONEL has a fast onset of action with fracture (bone breakage) reduction within six months.

- **BONIVA (ibandronate).** Dose: 150 mg monthly by mouth (or by injection every three months). BONIVA is only FDA approved to reduce the risk of vertebral (spine) fractures, and you must wait at least 60 minutes prior to eating or drinking other beverages if you are on monthly oral BONIVA.

- **FOSAMAX (alendronate sodium).** Dose: 70 mg and 35 mg weekly (the 70 mg dose is also available in liquid form). FOSAMAX has been FDA approved to reduce the risk of vertebral (spine) and hip fractures.

- **FOSAMAX PLUS D (alendronate).** Dose: 70 mg plus 2,800 IU of vitamin D or 70 mg plus 5,600 IU of vitamin D weekly in one pill. Alendronate is now available in generic form, but for the reasons listed in chapter 11, I do not favor the generics.

- **RECLAST (zoledronic acid).** Dose: 5 mg intravenous, yearly. his agent has been used for years in the form of Zometa to treat cancer patients with abnormal calcium levels, but in 2007, it was officially approved to treat for postmenopausal osteoporosis and Paget's disease and, in 2008, was approved to reduce the risk of fractures in persons who had sustained a low trauma hip fracture. For persons with any gastrointestinal intolerance to the oral bisphosphonates, or anyone who simply wants the convenience of a once yearly infusion (over a 15-minute time frame), this is a nice addition to the treatment of osteoporosis. In the HORIZON recurrent fracture trial (involving both men and women who had had surgery to repair a fractured hip), those who received the RECLAST had a *lower* death rate than those who did not.

For any patients finishing up a two-year course of FORTEO (injectable PTH) or for any older patient on multiple medications who may forget to take even a monthly bone pill, I recommend RECLAST. For patients on Medicare, it may be more cost-effective for them to receive Reclast as it doesn't affect the Medicare Part D "doughnut hole" (a gap in prescription coverage). RECLAST is also the only osteoporosis agent that has shown mortality reduction in older persons who have already broken a bone. If you are going to receive Reclast via an IV, I recommend kidney function, calcium, and vitamin D levels be checked (as for any patient starting on a bisphosphonate). In addition, you need to be well hydrated and talk to your doctor about taking oral Tylenol (acetaminophen) or Motrin/Advil (ibuprofen) the day before, the day of, and the day after the infusion to reduce the risk of flulike symptoms. Women who have already taken an oral bisphosphonate do not seem to have the risk for symptoms, but in any event, you might want to take Tylenol or Motrin/Advil to prevent these symptoms.

Note: Only estrogen, ACTONEL, FOSAMAX, and RECLAST have been proven to reduce the risk of spinal and hip fractures, so they are the ones I recommend most frequently for my patients who need complete skeletal protection. EVISTA, Calcitonin and BONIVA have not been shown to reduce the risk of hip fractures.

Bisphosphonates are usually well tolerated, but they can be associated with some gastrointestinal upset. It's important for any woman on bisphosphonates to take calcium at a different time than the bisphosphonate because bisphosphonates are not well absorbed from the stomach. Any other item in the stomach (besides plain water) will inhibit the absorption of the medicine, which then goes through your intestines to be literally flushed down the toilet, instead of going to your bones, where it's needed.

What's All This I Hear About Midlife Jaw Problems?

Recently news stories have focused on osteonecrosis of the jaw (ONJ). This has been reported primarily in patients with myeloma or other cancers who are undergoing chemotherapy or radiation treatments and who have poor dental status and in those receiving intravenous bisphosphonates.

Just as the media have promoted "hormone hysteria," there has been some "jaw necrosis hysteria" as well. I'm disturbed when a patient tells me that her dentist told her to "choose between your teeth and your hips." This is absurd. It's also another reason that it's important to find a women's health physician who can evaluate your whole health, consider your family history, and determine the best individualized regimen for your bone health.

Actually, some research shows that, like estrogen, ACTONEL may be good for the gums and teeth. A study at Case Western Reserve University reported that compared to postmenopausal women who receive no bone therapy, postmenopausal women who take ACTONEL can see improvements in the health of their teeth and gums. Certainly, this area requires more study, and it is one area that I am involved in researching.

Furthermore, in the HORIZON Pivotal Fracture Trial, there was no increase in ONJ in the postmenopausal women receiving yearly RECLAST through an IV, compared to the women receiving placebo injections.

Only a handful of cases of ONJ have been reported in which oral bisphosphonates were taken by otherwise healthy postmenopausal women. The minute risk of ONJ has been blown out of proportion by the media.

Calcitonin

Calcitonin is a protein taken by injection or nasal spray. It is a naturally occurring hormone that helps regulate calcium and bone metabolism. Therefore, it can slow bone loss, increase spinal bone density, and relieve fracture pain. Calcitonin is recommended only for women more than five years beyond menopause. (It has not been studied in younger women.) No reduction in hip fractures has been seen with calcitonin, and it is generally used only after other agents have been tried. Overall, calcitonin is a weaker bone option compared to the other bone agents; however, in patients with spinal canal stenosis or pain from a recent spinal compression fracture, an analgesic, pain-relieving beneficial effect is sometimes seen.

Calcitonin is administered by one squirt in one nostril daily. Brand names include MIACALCIN, CALCIMAR, and FORTI-CAL; the latter tends to be the least expensive of the calcitonin sprays.

Hormone Therapy

Hormone therapy is an FDA-approved option for osteoporosis prevention and management. For menopausal women, HT is a good choice to prevent or alleviate the increased rate of bone loss, since it replenishes some of the lost estrogen. HT is also recommended for postmenopausal women who either began menopause early or have menopausal symptoms.

If low bone density is your primary problem and you don't need the additional benefits of hormone therapy to relieve menopause symptoms, you should discuss other options with your physician. HT might not be the answer for you. Each woman must be evaluated on an individual basis.

The estrogen (PREMARIN) and estrogen-progestin components of the Women's Health Initiative trials showed reduction of all types of fractures in the women taking hormone therapy. This is impressive, since the group of women who participated in the study were not determined to be at high risk for osteoporosis. Thus, estrogen is the *only* agent shown to reduce risks of all types of fractures in women of varying bone density levels.

The Latest Options

MENOSTAR. This is a very low-dose (0.014 mg) estradiol patch, replaced weekly. In general, as women get older, particularly once they've reached the age of 60, the amount of estrogen in hormone therapy should be reduced because there is an increased risk of stroke (approximately 1 out of 1,000 women over the age of 60 taking full-dose estrogen), just as there is a small but definite increased risk of stroke in women who use hormonal contraception, such as the birth control pill.

MENOSTAR may be a good option for women over age 60 who no longer have hot flashes but have osteopenia and who want to prevent further bone loss without taking other agents like the bisphosphonates.

It's important to note that dosage must be individualized. However, if women taking this low-dose therapy experience recurring hot flashes or bone loss, they may need more estrogen than this option can provide. Still, many women can use a very low dose of estrogen such as Menostar and do well.

Another advantage of Menostar is that a progestogen needs to be added only once or twice a year. Less exposure to progestogen means a decreased risk of breast cancer and blood clots, since risk increases with exposure.

Remember that if a woman has a uterus, she may still need to take progesterone to protect it. A woman whose uterus was not removed during hysterectomy increases her risk of endometrial cancer if she takes estrogen without progesterone. This is because when estrogen is not balanced by progesterone, it can cause an overgrowth of cells in the uterus. Progesterone protects the endometrium from this tissue overgrowth.

However, when a woman takes a very low dose of estrogen, such as Menostar, she needs to take much less progesterone as well. Therefore, she receives the benefit of estrogen without the risks that come with taking too much progestin.

Women whose uteruses were removed during hysterectomy do not generally need to use a progestin.

Raloxifene. EVISTA (the brand name for raloxifene) is taken daily (dose: 60 mg) with or without food.

EVISTA is a selective estrogen receptor modulator (SERM). SERMS (now referred to as "estrogen agonists-estrogen antagonists") work on some but not all estrogen receptors. Raloxifene acts like estrogen on the bone but does not stimulate the breast or the uterus. (However, EVISTA does not treat menopause symptoms like hot flashes or dry vagina.)

This option may be appealing to postmenopausal women with osteopenia who no longer have hot flashes, who are concerned about potential breast risks associated with long-term estrogen-progestin HT, but who still want to reduce their risk of spine fractures as well as their risk for invasive breast cancer. As of 2007, EVISTA was FDA approved to reduce the risk of postmenopausal estrogen receptor positive breast cancer.

Raloxifene has cholesterol benefits as well. However, in the RUTH (Raloxifene Use for the Heart) trial, women with or at high risk for heart disease or diabetes did not show reduction in their risk of heart disease while taking raloxifene. These women did not experience an overall increased risk of stroke as a result of taking raloxifene, but women who had a stroke during the time they were taking the raloxifene had both an increased risk of stroke death.

The good news is that several other large trials besides RUTH have shown a reduction in breast cancer in women who take raloxifene, including the Multiple Outcomes of Raloxifene Evaluation (MORE) trial, which studied women with osteoporosis, and the Study of Tamoxifen and Raloxifene (STAR) trial, which studied women at increased risk for breast cancer.

Parathyroid Hormone. Teriparatide (brand name FORTEO) is a form of parathyroid hormone (PTH). The major hormone that regulates calcium levels in the blood, PTH is produced by the parathyroid glands, located next to the thyroid at the base of the neck. Another injectable form of PTH, called PREOS, may become available and will not need to be refrigerated like FORTEO.

FORTEO is an anabolic agent, which means that it actually stimulates new bone formation and increases bone density.

This treatment involves daily injection with a very small needle for eighteen to twenty-four months. Because of its expense and the need for injections, FORTEO is generally not a first line of treatment. However, parathyroid hormone is a very exciting option, particularly when other treatments don't work and women continue to fracture bones and/or have such severe low bone density that they need to build up bone. Bear in mind that once these injectable treatments are stopped, maintenance therapies are necessary to protect new bone.

In general, we don't use medications like FOSAMAX at the same time as a parathyroid hormone because it blunts the parathyroid's effects. However, they can be used sequentially. Also, estrogen and EVISTA can be used at the same time as parathyroid treatment, and the therapies appear to be additive.

So, women with menopause symptoms who are on estrogen but have severe osteoporosis might want to add FORTEO. Women who have been taking EVISTA but have fractured a bone may want to remain on EVISTA to reduce their risk of breast cancer while adding FORTEO to build bone.

Women who have Paget's disease or who have had radiation exposure are not candidates for this agent.

Stronium Ranelate. Strontium ranelate (PROTELOS) is a periodic element used in Europe in postmenopausal women to reduce the risk of fracture, but it is not available in the United States.

If I Feel Better, Can I Just Stop Using Bone Therapy?

Always consult a physician about bone therapy. Never stop taking recommended treatments without a discussion with your physician. I stress this point because you won't feel "progress" while taking these treatments. You won't notice that your bones are getting stronger or weaker, but they certainly can get weaker without the right treatment.

Supplements

The most effective way to prevent osteoporosis is to establish healthy habits early on. It's never too late to help bones the old-fashioned way, by drinking milk fortified with vitamin D3 and eating calcium-rich foods. Postmenopausal women over age 55 or women who are not on estrogen should consume 1,500 mg of calcium every day. Younger women or women who have had kidney stones should consume about 1,000 to 1,200 mg calcium citrate per day.

If you can't get the proper amounts through your daily diet, then supplements are an accessible, relatively safe choice. As always, consult your physician before beginning a supplement routine.

Calcium

I recommend calcium citrate supplements because the body absorbs them more easily and you can take them without food. They are more expensive than calcium carbonate. Either option is a step toward better bone health. Be careful not to consume more than 2,000 mg of calcium each day; excess consumption can increase the risk of kidney stones.

When considering how you take your calcium, keep in mind that your body can only absorb 500 mg of calcium at a time. Like a sponge that gets saturated and can't take in any more liquid,

Calcium in Your Cart

Fortify your grocery cart—and your bones—with calcium-rich foods. Here are some best bets:

- Almonds
- Blackstrap molasses
- Breads made with fortified flour
- Broccoli
- Canned fish (sardines, salmon)
- Cheese and other dairy foods
- Collards
- Dried beans
- Enriched orange juice (which can be fortified with calcium and vitamin D)
- Fortified cereals
- Kale
- Low-fat yogurt
- Milk
- Salmon (with bones)
- Spinach

If you're lactose intolerant, you may still be able to digest certain yogurts and hard cheeses. Try lactose-free dairy products and choose other lactose-free foods high in calcium from this list. Another solution is to purchase lactase (the enzyme that digests lactose), which can help your body digest dairy products.

your gut gets "saturated" with calcium. If you take your daily recommended dosage of 2,000 mg all at once, only 500 mg will be absorbed. Your body will excrete the rest.

Calcium levels should be monitored in those women who are on medications such as injectable FORTEO. If there are problems with calcium balance, your physician should obtain blood tests and urine calcium levels.

If you have kidney stones and are worried about worsening them by taking extra calcium, calcium citrate may pose a lower risk of kidney stones than calcium carbonate, which was shown in the Women's Health Initiative to increase slightly the risk of kidney stones. (Many of the participants were probably taking calcium in addition to the calcium provided in the study.)

Women who already have kidney stones will not reduce their risk of getting them again by cutting down on calcium. So if you have kidney stones, talk to your physician, use calcium citrate, maintain good hydration, and see whether your doctor thinks it would be a good idea to collect your urine for twenty-four hours to see how much calcium is being excreted.

Vitamin D

Vitamin D helps absorb calcium, so choose a calcium supplement that contains both. Take 1,000 IU of vitamin D3 each day. Vitamin D deficiency is very common, particularly in northern latitudes such as northeast Ohio, where I practice. For many women, this is due to insufficient intake. If a woman has unexplained vitamin D and/or iron deficiency, she should be evaluated for malabsorption and celiac disease.

Preventing Bone Loss

Along with the steps mentioned above, you can prevent bone loss by engaging in these measures:

- **Avoid certain medications.** Steroids, some breast cancer treatments, drugs used to treat seizures, blood thinners, and thyroid medications can increase the rate of bone loss. If you are taking any of these medicines, you need to be monitored more closely than usual.

- **Limit alcohol; stop smoking.** Your body makes less estrogen when you smoke, and too much alcohol can damage bones, although a moderate amount of alcohol (three to five drinks per week) is not harmful.

- **Participate in sensible weight-bearing exercises.** Weight-bearing activities force your muscles to work against gravity. Try walking, hiking, stair-climbing, or jogging. Lower-impact exercises may be preferred by some women, who may choose to lift weights or participate in water aerobics. Aim for thirty minutes of regular exercise three to four days a week, or at least every other day. Daily exercise for one hour is ideal. My motto is that exercise is the only sure-fire anti-aging remedy we have.

   For women who have definite osteoporosis and who are engaged in activities that may result in a fall (such as skiing), there are specific hip-pad protectors that can be worn comfortably under clothing. If you have osteoporosis, beware of such slip-and-fall risks as electrical cords, rugs, and slippery surfaces. A fall could result in a bone fracture. Another good idea is to install assistive devices if necessary.

Your bone health is manageable, if you just know where to start.

Chapter 13

Abnormal Bleeding and What to Do About It

H ere's an interesting question: What constitutes abnormal bleeding when you're entering menopause and expecting changes in your normal menstrual pattern anyway?

It's hard to say. Changes in menstrual bleeding are natural during perimenopause. Your flow may be heavier, you may have spotting, and the time between your periods may be longer or shorter.

Linda

It has been years since Linda has worn white pants or a white skirt. As she moved through her 40s, her menstrual periods got heavier and heavier, to the point that two supersized tampons and a thick pad were barely enough. She visited her local gynecologist, who was rushing to sign her up for a hysterectomy. Her mother and sister had hysterectomies, so Linda figured that she would probably need one, too. But she was concerned that she wasn't offered any other options, so she decided to seek another opinion.

When I saw Linda, I measured blood count and thyroid function because low thyroid can cause heavy periods. Despite taking iron daily, she was anemic with a hemoglobin of 8 (the normal is 12). When I asked her if she was craving things that were not food, she sheepishly admitted that she would chew on aluminum can tops. The medical term for this is pica, and it is a sign of low iron. Her general practitioner had already ordered a GI workup, and she had undergone an upper endoscopy and colonoscopy to check her intestinal tract and make sure there was no other sign of blood loss. Her GI workup was normal; however, I discovered that she had not been tested for Von Willebrand disease (an inherited bleeding disorder often overlooked as a medical cause of heavy periods) or platelet defects. I was suspicious about this because she had bled very heavily with a routine dental extraction as well as during her one vaginal delivery. She had nearly required a blood transfusion after she gave birth but noted that her periods were much better controlled when she was on the birth control pill.

The Von Willebrand panel came back, and indeed she did have mild Von Willebrand disease syndrome. She was treated with DDAVP-nasal spray for her bleeding disorder. I still had Linda scheduled for an office hysteroscopy, to make sure that we weren't missing any structural problems, even though her prior endometrial biopsies and pelvic ultrasounds by her local gynecologist were normal. As it turns out, she did have a very small polyp that was easily removed through the hysteroscope with in an in-and-out procedure. With the treatment of her mild Von Willebrand and the removal of this polyp, her blood count has returned to normal and she has not required hysterectomy.

This chapter is about abnormal bleeding and its treatments, including but not limited to hysterectomy. Once again, it's mostly about choice. I want to be sure that if a hysterectomy is recommended to you, you've understood your diagnosis and investigated all your options. Too many women aren't informed of their therapeutic choices.

How Do I Know What's "Abnormal?"

Remember that earlier we defined menopause as not having had a period for twelve months? We also noted that any bleeding after six months without a period should be checked out. Abnormal bleeding is bleeding that occurs any time after you've stopped having periods for six months or more.

Variations in bleeding can range from light spotting to a discharge comparable to a menstrual period. In severe cases, women may flood, leaking blood through tampons or sanitary napkins. Women who have had this experience are afraid to leave the house to run errands and worry about whether they'll have an accident at work.

Abnormal bleeding can be an isolated incident for some women, but for others it's a recurring situation. Sometimes abnormal bleeding is accompanied by abdominal pain, lower-back pain, pelvic cramping, and bowel or bladder problems. Bleeding can sometimes signify serious health concerns, which we'll identify below.

Should I Be Worried About Bleeding After the Onset of Menopause?

Abnormal bleeding from the uterus, vagina, or cervix is scary. The first concerns that come to mind are pelvic cancers, such as uterine or cervical cancer. Panic strikes. In most cases, however, women experience abnormal bleeding for benign and/or easily treated hormonal reasons. (And actually, uterine and ovarian cancers can present with no bleeding at all.)

So don't panic if you have abnormal bleeding and try not to jump to conclusions that the cause is cancer or a life-threatening illness. However, do see a women's health doctor to get checked out.

• • • *Fast Fact* • • •

Sometimes a uterine infection will cause spotting
or abnormal bleeding. This is one reason I tell
women not to douche, as it can shoot bacteria
into the uterus and cause a low-grade infection that
can result in abnormal bleeding. If you feel the need to
douche, use over the counter repHresh gel instead.

• • •

Is Hysterectomy the Only Treatment for Abnormal Bleeding?

Prior to contemplating hysterectomy, any woman who has unexplained causes of heavy bleeding should be evaluated for an underlying mild bleeding disorder or a subclinical thyroid condition, even if she has a known fibroid or endometrial polyp.

Many women in my practice who suffer from severe menopausal symptoms have had hysterectomies needlessly. I ask them how they are faring, and they say they feel violated. No one told them there were other ways to treat fibroids besides taking out their insides. The side effects are physical and emotional. They feel cheated. (Of course, many women are thrilled not to deal with a monthly period or worry about a surprise pregnancy. After a hysterectomy, many women make a smooth transition into menopause.)

My goal is to help you understand the surgical solutions to various types of abnormal bleeding and make sure that you know how to get information from a knowledgeable physician who can steer you toward the option that's right for you.

Many times there are nonhysterectomy alternatives. For example, for heavy bleeding, if the evaluation is negative, we will consider insertion of an intrauterine system, the Mirena IUS (a contraceptive) because the constant local application of a progestin will slow down the menstrual flow or even stop the flow.

However, in cases where the uterus is very large (to the belly button or the size of a four-month pregnancy) because of uterine fibroids, particularly if the uterus is pressing on other internal organs like the kidney, a hysterectomy is usually needed. This decision is only made after careful consideration.

Here are some important questions that are frequently skipped when a hysterectomy is suggested:

- Do you really need a hysterectomy?

- Did your physician explain noninvasive procedures for treating benign conditions like uterine fibroids, endometriosis, or pelvic prolapse?

- Are you aware that there are options other than removing your uterus and ovaries, which sends the body into abrupt, surgical menopause?

Investigating the Cause

Abnormal vaginal bleeding after menopause can have many causes, including infection, inflammation, injury, or abnormal growths, whether benign or malignant. These can also cause bleeding that is erratic.

Specifically, potential causes for abnormal bleeding include:

- **Hormone imbalance.** Too much estrogen and/or not enough progesterone and/or absence of regular ovulation.

- **Atrophy.** Excessive thinness of the lining of the uterus (the endometrium) as well as a lack of estrogen can lead to vaginal thinning, which can lead to vaginal bleeding.

- **Uterine fibroids.** These are noncancerous growths, especially the submucosal type (fibroids that develop on the inner side of the uterus), which can press on the endometrium.

- **Endometriosis.** The endometrium is the lining of the uterus. The growth of endometrial tissue in other parts of the body is called endometriosis.

- **Anovulatory bleeding.** This is bleeding that is caused by lack of regular ovulation. It's responsible for 70 percent of all abnormal uterine bleeding.

- **Uterine infection.** This can occur spontaneously or be from a sexually transmitted infection.

- **Endometrial hyperplasia (tissue overgrowth).** The uterine lining thickens without shedding; overgrown tissue is a breeding ground for abnormal cells (and a possible precursor to uterine cancer). If you have "stypia" this is a concern and a precursor to endometrial cancer.

- **Cystic glandular hyperplasia.** In this situation, there is too much uterine lining, but endometrial cells are generally normal.

- **Adenomatous hyperplasia.** This is a more advanced stage of hyperplasia. The endometrial cells are larger but still benign.

- **Atypical adenomatous hyperplasia.** This is severe hyperplasia. A small area or the entire lining of the endometrium is consumed by abnormal cells that are not necessarily benign. It is generally treated as an early cancer requiring hysterectomy.

- **Uterine cancer (endometrial carcinoma).** This requires a complete hysterectomy. It's usually completely curable if diagnosed early. Please don't delay about seeing a women's health physician if you have any abnormal bleeding.

Which Tests Should I Have?

If you have abnormal bleeding, a medical evaluation is the first order of business. It should include a pelvic exam, Pap test, and HPV DNA test.

Next, your physician will investigate the bladder and colon for infection. You may need a colonoscopy to rule out bowel problems or any precursors to colon cancer, as sometimes women aren't sure if they are having bleeding from the rectum or vagina.

Assuming your evaluation is clear so far, there are other tests a knowledgeable physician can make to determine the cause of bleeding and whether a hysterectomy or another treatment is necessary.

D & C (Dilation and Curettage). Until relatively recently, gynecologists have depended on D & C procedures to "clean out" the uterus. A big drawback to D & Cs are that they are done "blind." A tool is inserted into the uterus through the cervix, and the area is literally scraped. The doctor can easily miss fibroids, abnormal cell growths, or small polyps.

A D & C procedure, or even two, won't necessarily control bleeding because the doctor may not remove the actual cause of the problem if she can't see it.

Fortunately, there are now more modern options.

Hysteroscopy. A lighted scope is inserted through the vagina and cervix into the uterus. The instrument can be used to examine the endometrium, as well as to collect a biopsy sample and guide minimally invasive surgery to remove any abnormal growths without having to remove the entire uterus.

The procedure takes thirty minutes and can be performed during an office visit. If polyps or fibroids are to be removed, it's done in a surgical suite with some anesthesia.

If you need hysteroscopy or SIS (see below), ask your doctor whether you should take 200 mg of Cytotec (misoprostol) orally to dilate the cervix. This could make the procedure easier on you.

Transvaginal Pelvic Ultrasound. A small ultrasound device is inserted into the vagina to produce a picture of the uterus and pelvic structures. This test determines whether uterine fibroids are present and whether the uterine lining is too thick (generally in postmenopausal women, 5mm to 4mm or less is reassuring). An ultrasound also allows the doctor to look at both of the ovaries.

Saline Infusion Sonography (SIS). Sterile saline (saltwater) is passed into the uterus through a small, soft plastic tube. Infused saline separates uterus walls so the sonogram can identify irregularities of the inner uterine wall. (Regular ultrasounds often cannot capture these specific images.) Polyps in the uterus or localized thickening can be identified this way.

Uterine Fibroids

Uterine fibroids are nodules (small collections of muscle tissue) made up of smooth muscle cells and fibrous connective tissue that develop within the wall of the uterus. Medically, they are called uterine leiomyomata (the singular is leiomyoma).

Fibroids may grow as a single nodule or in clusters and may range in size from 1 mm to more than 20 cm (8 inches) in diameter. They may grow within the wall of the uterus, or they may project into the interior cavity or toward the outer surface of the uterus. When they grow on stems projecting from the surface of the uterus they're called "pedunculated."

Most women with uterine fibroids will never know they have them since symptoms do not always present. But some women *will* have symptoms, which can include the following:

- Abnormal bleeding that mimics a heavy period, longer periods, or bleeding between periods
- A sudden, heavy flow after not having a period for several months
- Pelvic pain, including pain during sex
- Lower back pain that doesn't go away
- Abdominal pain
- Urinary or bowel problems

Are Fibroids Painful?

Fibroids of small to moderate size that do not cause symptoms and are confirmed as benign by a knowledgeable physician do not need to be surgically removed. They may never cause symptoms or be painful, and after menopause, they're likely to shrink and go away.

However, when fibroids grow large, they can push on organs like the kidneys and cause pressure in the back and abdomen. In severe cases, clusters of fibroids can grow so large that they outstrip their blood supply, causing the attached part of the muscle to die. When this happens, the uterus and fibroids both shrink, causing a muscle attack and severe pain in the pelvic region. This situation can lead to the need for an emergency hysterectomy.

Fibroids cause pressure in the back and abdomen when they grow large and push on organs like kidneys.

How Are Fibroids Treated?

Once your physician confirms that the reason for your abnormal bleeding, pelvic discomfort, or chronic pain is indeed a fibroid (or several of them), she will discuss a few treatment options with you. In addition to diagnostic office hysteroscopy followed by therapeutic operative hysteroscopic resection of a fibroid, options include open surgical myomectomy to remove only the fibroid, if it isn't accessible via the hysteroscope, or hysterectomy to remove fibroids and the uterus. On rare occasions during a complete hysterectomy, ovaries are also removed. (We'll talk more about hysterectomy, and whether it is necessary, later in this chapter.)

More and more, physicians are beginning to realize that uterine fibroids may not require any intervention or limited treatment at most. For a woman with uterine fibroids that aren't causing symptoms, the best therapy may be watchful waiting.

Myomectomy Options. Depending on the size, location, and number of fibroids, your physician may recommend one of these surgeries to remove just fibroids. These surgeries fall under the umbrella of operations called "myomectomy," meaning excision of a myoma (a tumor consisting of muscle tissue).

These options are favored over hysterectomy, which eliminates a woman's ability to give birth. (You might not be interested in childbearing, but if you develop fibroids while you're still planning a family or if you simply want to avoid major gynecological surgery, you need to know all of your choices for fibroid treatment.)

Before myomectomy, Lupron injections are often used to shrink the size of the fibroid. Lupron is a gonadotropin-releasing hormone analogue (GnRH analogue) that decreases the body's production of estrogen to menopausal levels. It is not a long-term treatment, because it puts a woman into temporary menopause, but it is helpful in sorting out potential diagnoses and affords some temporary treatment.

Types of myomectomy include the following:

- **Hysteroscopy.** Described on page 233, hysteroscopic resection is used to remove fibroids on the inner wall of the uterus.

- **Laparoscopy.** One or more small incisions are made in the abdomen to remove at most one or two fibroids that are up to two inches in diameter and growing on the outside of the uterus.

- **Laparotomy.** A larger incision is made in the abdomen to remove large fibroids, multiple fibroids, or deep-rooted growths from the uterine wall.

- **UFE or UAE.** Uterine fibroid embolization, also known as uterine artery embolization, is a minimally invasive approach to treating fibroids by blocking the arteries that supply blood flow to them. The process involves placing a catheter in the uterine arteries by making a small incision at the top of the leg. A needle is used to enter the artery and provide access for the catheter. Then, guided by X-rays, small particles are injected into the arteries feeding the fibroids, resulting in their blockage.

    Lupron should not be used prior to UFE because it can affect the blood flow to the uterus, and the radiologist injecting the particles into the uterine arteries needs to get a full picture of that blood flow.

Endometriosis

Characterized by chronic pelvic pain and sometimes by abnormal bleeding, endometriosis is the growth of endometrial tissue in other parts of the body besides the uterus. Hot spots for endometrial growths include the abdominal cavity, ovaries, fallopian tubes, bowels, and the outer surface of the uterus.

These growths are essentially displaced uterine wall tissue, and they act as such. They want to shed each month just as the uterus does during a menstrual period, and they do. The bleeding sometimes causes pain. And when scar tissue develops over these lesions, it can interfere with organ functions. For example, when tissue blocks the fallopian tubes, a woman can become infertile. She may experience few symptoms except this and wonder why she cannot get pregnant.

Symptoms of endometriosis vary widely and can include the following:

- Pelvic pain/and or painful intercourse
- Infertility
- Abnormal periods
- Nausea and/or dizziness
- Exhaustion
- Bladder problems
- Frequent infections
- Painful bowel movements or irritable bowels
- Aching back, abdomen, and pelvic region
- Other stomach problems

How Is Endometriosis Treated?

Laparoscopic surgery and hormone therapies, such as Lupron shots, for short-term alleviation are all options.

Laparoscopic surgery is the most common procedure for removing mild to moderate endometriosis. Instead of using a large abdominal incision, the surgeon inserts a lighted viewing instrument. (Laparoscopic surgery is described earlier in this chapter on page 237.)

Pregnancy sometimes improves endometriosis.

Thiamine has been shown to reduce menstrual cramps when they're a problem.

Identifying and Treating Adenomyosis

Endometriosis is bleeding on the outside of the uterus, and adenomyosis is bleeding on the inside. Adenomyosis is a form of endometriosis characterized by the invasive, usually benign, growth of tissue into uterine muscle.

How Is Adenomyosis Treated?

If you have unexplained pain and diagnostic testing indicates the cause is not fibroids, adenomyosis could be the culprit, especially if you've had a C-section. You could actually be bleeding inside the uterus muscles.

The best way to identify adenomyosis is with a pelvic MRI. Another option is to shut down the period (and bleeding) using continuous birth control or a shot of Lupron, which puts a woman in medical menopause. When bleeding stops, symptoms should stop. If symptoms flare up again when you stop taking the birth control and Lupron, then adenomyosis may be the diagnosis.

Adenomyosis is conventionally treated by hysterectomy, but nonsurgical procedures can also remedy the problem. Many times, insertion of the MIRENA IUS will decrease bleeding and cramps. It can be effective for five to seven years while providing contraception (if needed) as well. I think any woman contemplating either a tubal ligation for sterilization or a hysterectomy for menstrual disorder should first consider the MIRENA IUS.

Adenomyosis or Fibroids?

Fibroids are generally self-contained growths, while adenomyosis is overgrowth of tissue between layers of the uterine muscle wall.

What If My Doctor Can't Determine the Cause of My Abnormal Bleeding?

After ruling out infection, cancer, endometrial polyps, and uterine fibroids, a women's health physician can "ablate," or physically destroy, the uterine lining so that it won't become thick and shed in a procedure called "endometrial ablation."

This procedure is only appropriate if

- you are still bleeding and the cause is not a bleeding disorder;
- you do not want to take hormones continuously to suppress your period; and
- you do not desire any pregnancies.

Endometrial ablation is not the first line of treatment. Women under age 40 should avoid ablation, and the procedure usually can be performed only twice before a woman will require a hysterectomy. It's a good option for women in their late 40s who are close to menopause and are bothered by menstrual flooding.

Other options for treating heavy periods include these:

- **MECLOMEN.** This and other nonsteroidal anti-inflammatory drugs (NSAIDS) slow down menstrual flow and reduce or stop cramping.

- **MIRENA IUS.** This product contains levonorgestrel and is associated with lighter periods.
- **SEASONALE or SEASONIQUE.** These give you twelve weeks of hormone contraception with a period "once a season."
- **LYBREL.** Comprises 365 days of active pills/hormonal contraception with no placebo breaks.

Hysterectomy: Become Informed

Unfortunately, many women who bleed abnormally are treated with hysterectomies, and that's no treat. A woman really needs to be counseled before making a decision that will change her body forever. Here are some questions she should consider:

- Are you ready to lose your uterus?
- Do you plan on having more children?
- Are you prepared for menopause and the severe side effects that affect some women who have full hysterectomies?

Depending on your reason for considering hysterectomy, your feelings about the procedure will vary. If your mother had ovarian cancer and you want a full hysterectomy (removal of the ovaries and uterus), this procedure may be the only way for you to gain peace of mind. But there are consequences to losing your ovaries. For many women, it isn't worth it. The situation is analogous to that of a woman whose mother had breast cancer and who learns that she too has the BRCA breast cancer gene. While one woman might choose to have her breast removed (mastectomy or the newer nipple-sparing mastectomy) as a preventive measure, another might not want to go through such a procedure, preferring to reduce her risk of breast and ovarian cancer by having only her ovaries removed.

The point is, your physician should outline the pros and cons so that you can decide. If your physician is not engaging you in this discussion, you need to seek a knowledgeable professional in women's health who will. You deserve to know the benefits and consequences of such serious surgeries. And today, if you prefer an alternative to hysterectomy, there are more options than ever before.

Hysterectomy is the surgical removal of the uterus, and women undergo this procedure for a variety of reasons: gynecological conditions, including childbirth complications; cancer; and abnormal bleeding due to fibroids or endometriosis.

There are three types of hysterectomy, and your physician should discuss these options and what is most appropriate for your case:

- **Partial hysterectomy.** This surgical removal of the uterus may or may not include leaving the cervix in place. This is the most common procedure.

- **Complete hysterectomy.** This involves removal of both uterus and cervix.

- **Radical (total) hysterectomy.** This involves removal of the uterus, cervix, ovaries, structures that support the uterus, and sometimes the lymph nodes. This aggressive procedure is used in response to endometriosis and some cancers.

When Is Hysterectomy Not Necessary?

Many cases do not necessarily warrant hysterectomy. In these instances, the choice is yours. Abnormal bleeding does not mean that you need to give up your uterus. A fibroid is no reason to undergo hysterectomy. If you're diagnosed with a benign condition, your next stop doesn't need to be medical menopause.

Exceptions to this are if the fibroid is cancerous, rapidly growing, or causing severe pain and inflammation.

If your physician suggests a hysterectomy for the following conditions, get a second opinion, then a third—trust your judgment:

- Fibroids
- Uterine prolapse
- Endometriosis
- Ovarian cysts (benign)
- Severe premenstrual syndrome (PMS)
- Adenomyosis
- Heavy bleeding

When Is Hysterectomy Nonnegotiable?

When a woman carries a BRCA gene, which indicates a high risk for breast or ovarian cancer, complete hysterectomy or at least removal of both ovaries can be an important option after childbearing is completed. And when pelvic procedures fail to treat endometriosis, a full hysterectomy is in order.

Also, women who have cervical cancer need a hysterectomy that includes removal of the cervix. Uterine and ovarian cancers also require complete hysterectomy.

In each case, here are some implications that might influence your decision to get a full hysterectomy (removing ovaries, uterus, and cervix) or to remove only parts of the whole.

If You Have the BRCA Gene. You may choose to keep your uterus and have only the ovaries removed laparoscopically, but in my opinion, once the ovaries are gone and you enter surgical menopause, you then may have to take estrogen to control your symptoms. If you need estrogen and have a uterus, you need to take a progestogen to protect the uterus. And it may be the progestogens and not estrogen that, over the long term, increase the risk for breast cancer and blood clots.

Save the Cervix?

Generally speaking, the cervix is removed during the time of hysterectomy. But for some women, the cervix is an erogenous zone, and they may choose to keep it so that its removal doesn't change their sex lives. These are women who report sexual stimulation with "cervical tapping." In general, removing the cervix will not affect sexual function for the great majority of women.

Be aware that if you keep your cervix after hysterectomy, you still need to get a Pap test every two to three years and an HPV DNA test by age 30.

So if you're going to have both ovaries removed, I usually recommend removal of the uterus, too, even though this surgical procedure takes longer than one in which only the ovaries are removed.

If Pelvic Procedures Did Not Treat Your Endometriosis. In this circumstance, you may need to have the uterus, ovaries, and cervix removed.

If You're Under Age 65. Unless you're at a high risk for breast or ovarian cancer, I recommend that your ovaries not be removed during hysterectomy, because there is a survival advantage in keeping the ovaries.

So often there's more than one possibility for an appropriate treatment or procedure. Please be sure that you're fully informed and understand your choices. It truly is your body, your hormones, and your choice.

Conclusion

Your Body, Your Choices

Many women seek balance during midlife. Perhaps this is because menopause introduces so many hormone shifts and lifestyles changes that we simply need to find that balanced perspective. Our children mature. We find time to unwind from demanding professional lives, or perhaps we renew personal energy by beginning a new venture. We realize that as we mature, our spirits stay lively. Longevity, in many respects, is a choice.

All this makes midlife an ideal time to evaluate your life, to reflect on your past from a personal perspective. Look how far you've come! Midlife is also time to plan for the future. It's never too early or too late to focus on disease prevention, health promotion, and enhanced vitality.

The medical discipline of women's health has come a long way, too. We know more than ever before about hormonal health and ways to strike a balance in that arena. We continue to research the effects of new medications and treatments. We are learning ways to help women feel better, age better, and live better.

Of course, with all this learning and research, there may come new, unanswered questions, which perhaps can lead to confusion and fear. This calls for the big job of translating any partial truths and looking at the whole picture.

Because women are inundated with misleading messages, teasing out the facts is difficult. You must read the fine print. You must tune out the relatives and friends who discourage you from doing what's best for you. So many times, women tell me that other women have admonished them about their choices. "Why are you still on hormones if you're 65?" In return, I would ask, "Whose body is it anyway?"

Unfortunately, a significant portion of the medical community has adopted a similar unsupportive approach to treating women, largely, I believe, because of popular fear and overblown research. Whether the topic is breast-feeding, menstrual periods, hysterectomy, menopause, or birth control options, everyone wants to weigh in. This is harmful when women feel constricted by opinions that dismiss real options. In effect, we limit our choices because we hear out of context that something is "bad." "Hormones are bad." "Not breast-feeding is bad." "Taking birth control at age 50 is bad."

This mentality is damaging to women. It weighs heavily on a woman's personal decisions about her health and her body. Such pressure might just ruin her chance of striking the balance that is right for her. How can you feel at ease when so many voices are speaking out of turn? The voice you should listen to is your own. Remember: It truly is your body, your hormones, and your choices.

In chapter 13, when I was discussing hysterectomy procedures, I mentioned that you should seek a second opinion, maybe even a third, and then trust your gut. If you aren't getting answers from your doctor, find someone who will talk to you. If you feel as if the talk is just a quick pitch for a decision you're not comfortable with, start another discussion. Don't settle for "doctor's orders" if the instructions you're given limit your choices and don't take into account your personal needs, lifestyle, and preferences.

You are the authority on your health. Don't trust companies, books, or practices that sell "guaranteed" or "natural and risk-free" treatments for hot flashes, sexual difficulties, or any other symptom. If you're receiving conflicting advice from your otherwise trustworthy general practitioner (who is probably not a hormone expert), don't turn to those shady folks ready to test your saliva, take your money, and mix up unregulated hormones—seek out a NAMS-certified menopause health care provider through *www.menopause.org* or a well-respected women's health specialist.

Also, please take to heart the message that women deserve to look and feel good. Give yourself opportunities to look and feel better by learning about your options. Women have more choices today than ever before.

Remember too that women deserve to sleep well and don't need to suffer from menstrual flooding, mood problems, severe menopause symptoms, leaky bladder, or osteoporosis. Just because you're a woman, you don't have to be a martyr or a victim.

During midlife, you should look forward to vibrant years during which you feel comfortable in your own skin, confident in your decisions, and inspired by the possibilities of your second adulthood. Celebrate your accomplishments, measure your progress, and set some new goals.

The key to reaching them is keeping your good health and your options opened.

Acknowledgments

I thank my husband, Tom G. Thacker, II, and our three sons, Stetson, Emerson, and Grayson, who encouraged me to "write the book" and then to update the book. As my husband said, "Suzanne Somers's book is fiction, while this book is nonfiction." I am especially thankful to work with so many dedicated women and talented staff at the Cleveland Clinic Center for Specialized Women's Health.

Appendix 1

Preventive Care

Preventive care for women includes health screenings and immunizations. Here are some lists to help you prevent the most common problems plaguing midlife women.

General Preventive Care

- Breast cancer screening, starting at age 40, with yearly mammograms for all women. Best to get right after your period or after the progesterone regimen of cycled HT.

- Cervical cancer screening, starting at age 21 or three years after becoming sexually active—whichever comes first.

- Colorectal screening, starting at age 50 or sooner if you have a family history.

- Periodic screening for cholesterol (at least every five years), hypertension (yearly blood pressure checks), diabetes (blood sugars every three years), and osteoporosis (by menopause and every two to five years pending results), and thyroid disorders (TSH thyroid blood tests every five years or yearly if on thyroid hormone).

- Tetanus booster every ten years. Get the new tetanus booster Tdap (Adacel), which covers tetanus, diphtheria, and whooping cough (acellular pertussis), if you are under age 64 and have not received it.

- Flu vaccine every fall for women over age 50. For women who prefer to avoid a shot, FluMist nasal spray vaccine is now available.

- Women over age 60 (or younger, if they have chronic medical problems) should have the pneumonia vaccine PNEU-MOVAX. If you have had chickenpox but have not yet had shingles, get ZOSTAVAX, the shingles vaccine (check with your insurance company regarding coverage).

- Young girls and young women should consider the HPV vaccine Gardasil as well as the meningitis vaccine Menactra.

- Avoid certain medications. Steroids, some breast cancer treatments, drugs used to treat seizures, blood thinners, and thyroid medications can increase the rate of bone loss. If you are taking any of these medicines, you need to be monitored more closely than usual.

- Limit alcohol; stop smoking. Your body makes less estrogen when you smoke, and too much alcohol can damage bones, although a moderate amount of alcohol (three to five drinks per week) is not harmful.

- Wear a seat belt every time you're in a vehicle.

- Eat a healthy, nutritious, and colorful diet.

- Exercise daily—one hour is best.

- Create your living will and medical power of attorney.

Tests for Cervical and Gynecological Cancers

- HPV DNA testing (plus a ThinPrep Pap Test) is the new standard of care. It's very important for women with abnormal Paps and women over the age of 30.

- The American College of Obstetrics and Gynecology recommends HPV and Pap screening for cervical cancer in women age 30 and older. If both results are normal, they can reduce testing to every three years in healthy women. Women with HIV/AIDS need more frequent screens.

- If a woman has a positive result on HPV testing but a negative result on Pap testing, she should repeat both tests in six to twelve months.

- With increasing age, the likelihood increases that a positive HPV test will represent persistent disease. Only those who have persistent high-risk HPV infections are at risk for cervical cancer.

Breast-Imaging Options

- Digital mammography may be better for certain types of women, including those under age 50, who have very dense breasts and/or are premenopausal or perimenopausal.

- Other options for diagnostic imaging include breast ultrasound, dedicated breast MRI, and ductography. These options can be very helpful when a diagnosis is equivocal or in confirming a diagnosis.

Bio-identical and Bio-similar Hormone Therapy

- Bio-identical hormone therapy is catching the attention of women across the country. It simply means using hormones that are identical to human hormones.

- Bio-similar hormones are the hormones found in hormonal contraceptives and many standardized, well-studied hormone therapy prescriptions.

- Hormone therapy—including bio-similar therapy—is an important option for women. It remains the gold standard for minimizing menopause symptoms, treating changes in vitality, and maintaining and protecting bone strength.

- Hormone therapy can be successful when it's tailored to the individual woman.

- Women need to beware of the pitfalls of compounding pharmacies in which hormone doses are *not* standardized or regulated. (They're derived from synthesized hormones in a laboratory, and doses can vary.)

Get to Sleep, for Health's Sake

- Getting enough sleep helps prevent weight gain.

- Sleep disorders are common, and hormonal variations across a woman's life span are more likely to be diagnosed during midlife.

- When sleep apnea in postmenopausal women goes untreated, it's a risk for heart trouble, high blood pressure, and weight gain.

- Unusual sleep disorders, such as sleep-related eating disorder, can have serious consequences, including diabetes.

- Your sleep patterns will change as you age, especially during menopause. Tune in to your sleep concerns and discuss them with your doctor.

Osteoporosis: Building Bone Health in Midlife

- Osteoporosis is *not* a normal part of aging. It can be prevented and treated.

- Osteoporosis does not usually cause symptoms until you break a bone.

- Early awareness, regular weight-bearing exercise such as walking, and making sure that you take enough calcium and vitamin D are key. Talk to your doctor to make sure you are doing enough.

- Painful compression fractures of the spine—common in older women—are often caused by osteoporosis and can lead to deformity, such as loss of height and a humped back or "dowager's hump."

- Vertebroplasty and kyphoplasty are surgical treatments that may be considered for compression fractures to help relieve pain, restore some of the lost height, and correct the spinal deformity.

Keys to Healthy Joints

- Eat a healthy, balanced diet with brightly colored fruits and vegetables high in antioxidants. Get enough vitamin D—at least 1,000 IU to 2,000 IU daily.

- Reduce daily biomechanical stress, a common trigger for joint pain. Try exercises easy on the joints, such as swimming or water aerobics.

- Aim for thirty to sixty minutes of exercise daily.

- Lose excess weight. Even an extra five pounds places unnecessary stress on joints.

- Prevent exercise injuries. Warm up and stretch properly before and after exercise.

- Glucosamine may help reduce arthritis of the knee in postmenopausal women. Try 1,500 mg for at least two months before deciding whether it helps your joints.

Build a Better Memory

- The ability to learn and recall new information can be affected by a variety of factors, including normal aging, situational factors (stress or poor sleep), mood disorders, hormones, medications, and underlying medical problems.

- How hormone therapy affects memory is controversial. HT may be associated with cognitive benefits, but they seem to vary depending on the woman's age at the time HT is used.

- Lifestyle factors, mood disorders, and other medical variables are far more likely to result in significant memory difficulties than are normal hormonal changes.

- Maintaining a healthy lifestyle, reducing stress, exercising your brain, and working closely with a trusted physician to ensure optimal health will help you maintain memory function throughout your life.

Managing Mood Disorders

- Women are more prone to depression than men, particularly during times of hormone fluctuation.
- Treatment is available for hormone-related mood disorders.
- Depression is treatable.
- Psychotherapy and lifestyle changes are beneficial for the depressed woman.
- See a doctor to rule out medical causes for depression—check thyroid levels.

Acupuncture

- Acupuncture is an ancient healing art.
- Traditional thinking about why acupuncture works is based on a completely different understanding of the body's anatomy than we use in Western medicine. It is based on *qi* ("chee"), a person's life force, and the pathways, or "meridians," through which it flows.
- Studies show that acupuncture is safe and effective and that it releases endorphins and activates morphine receptors.
- Acupuncture affects the neurotransmitter chemicals in the brain that can influence mood and pain perception.

Prevent Stroke

- When a stroke occurs, *call 911 immediately.* Calling 911 is the best way to get urgent medical attention. Stroke is a "brain attack." The longer medical attention is withheld, the more brain tissue and, thus, brain function dies.

- Know the risk factors for stroke. Screening and treatment for medical conditions such as hypertension (high blood pressure), diabetes, high cholesterol, and heart disease are the best means to prevent stroke and heart attack.

- After talking to your doctor, consider taking a daily baby aspirin, especially if you're over age 65. Daily baby aspirin in women age 65 and older has been associated with a 30 percent decreased risk in stroke.

- Adopt a healthy lifestyle. Don't smoke and support family and friends who are trying to quit. Eat a healthy diet and keep your waistline under 35 inches. Exercise at least thirty to (preferably) sixty minutes daily.

Get Heart Smart

- Heart disease is the number one cause of death in women (and men).

- *Cardiovascular disease* is an overall term that includes five diseases: hypertension, coronary artery disease, congestive heart failure, stroke, and congenital heart disease (from birth).

- Symptoms women experience during a heart attack may differ from those men experience. In addition to chest pain or discomfort, women may have nausea/vomiting, shortness of breath, light-headedness, back or jaw pain, and simply more fatigue than usual.

- Risk factors for most types of heart disease include age, family history, high lipids (cholesterol and triglycerides), high blood pressure, diabetes, smoking, and obesity. (Diabetes and high triglycerides are especially potent risks for heart disease in women.)

Should You Purchase Medicines Online?

- Online pharmacies have become a mainstream, multibillion-dollar industry. Many medications are cheaper online, but not all are. Hidden costs include shipping and handling fees as well as online "cyber doctor" consultations necessary to obtain prescriptions.

- Online pharmacies often provide prescriptions for people despite clear contraindications.

- Medications purchased online may be expired, made in substandard facilities, or even counterfeit.

- Anyone using Internet pharmacies should be advised to choose only sites with a Verified Internet Pharmacy Practice Sites (VIPPS) logo, indicating that they have met standards set by the National Association of Boards of Pharmacy.

Appendix 2

Shared Medical Appointments

S cheduling a doctor's appointment can be a frustrating experience. Six-month backlogs and brief, ten-minute visits leave
many women feeling jilted at the office. Developing a relationship with a doctor during this brief window of time seems next
to impossible.

This is why a new concept, shared medical appointments
(SMA), offered through our Clinic Care Program, has been so beneficial to women in my practice. Shared visits do not take the place
of an initial, individual women's health evaluation but instead are
an enhancement of the medical services we provide.

After her private, one-on-one annual appointment, every
woman has the option of attending a shared follow-up visit if
she chooses. We host these sessions during set times each week.
Between ten and fourteen women may attend each session.

More hospitals and clinics are adopting this format as doctors
struggle to spend quality time with patients despite packed schedules and pressure to "move quickly" to keep up with heavy patient
loads. I have doctors, nurses, and administrators from around the
country come to observe my women's health shared visits. The
arrangement is beneficial for both doctors and patients; actually,
I find that many women learn more during these shared visits than
they do during one-on-one evaluations. Ask your health care provider whether this is an option for you.

One Woman's Experience

"My family thinks of me as the rock. They're right. I've been the listener, the advice giver, the loyal wife, the involved mother—you name it—for the last thirty years of my life. Menopause hit me hard. I'm actually relieved that my children are grown and don't live at home, because I can't imagine them seeing me so fragile. Sometimes I feel as if I'm just going to fall apart, and I usually do at least once a day.

"I've never been depressed, so I really had no idea why my body was responding so violently to 'the change.'

"I really needed this support. The medications helped me tremendously, but prescriptions alone weren't enough. My weaknesses were as much mental and spiritual as they were physical. Following my first shared visit, I made several individual appointments with the social worker. Now my days are much better, and when they aren't, I'm not so hard on myself."

Here's how they work. Before the session begins, each woman signs a confidentiality agreement and writes down any questions or concerns she'd like addressed during the appointment. I facilitate these appointments with a licensed behavioral health specialist, nurse, or other health professional who serves as a moderator.

At the beginning of a session, when some women shy away from discussing their medical histories openly, the moderator poses general questions to the group or discusses healthy habits, such as taking calcium in divided doses as well as at least 1,000 international units of vitamin D3 each day. She may ask: "Who has trouble sleeping? What do you do about it?"

The conversation that follows educates patients and begins helping them to feel comfortable talking with one another.

During this time, I speak with each person individually, review test results, follow up on prescriptions and recommendations, and address any individual concerns.

Our conference room is equipped with a comfortable couch and chairs, and we always have an assortment of beverages on hand. The setting facilitates advice and support from other women in a relaxed atmosphere.

The environment is a blend of the womanly support we all need during this time—the same "Do you know what I mean?" conversations that we have with our sisters and mothers—reinforced with access to medical and psychological care.

Using shared visits, patients can see me more often. And rather than cramming questions and concerns into a ten-minute individual session, women learn from each others' experiences and almost always leave the ninety-minute forums with some new "pearls" of wisdom and inspiration.

Are You a Candidate for a Shared Visit?

The shared-visit format isn't appropriate for every patient. Shared visits are not a replacement for individual office visits, and they are not appropriate for the following:

- Initial evaluations
- One-time consultations
- Complex medical procedures
- Treatment of acute infectious illnesses, vaginal discharge, a new breast lump, abnormal menstrual bleeding, or other urgent medical concerns
- Women who may be too sensitive to listen to other patients' issues

- Patients who have difficulty communicating or have a language barrier

Who Are the Best Candidates for Shared Visits?

For some women, a shared visit can have the impact of five one-on-one appointments with a physician. Even though I'm a woman and a physician, if I haven't experienced painful intercourse or used a prescription vaginal ring, I cannot offer the same perspective as another woman who can relate on a more direct level. I can offer medical support, while another woman can provide the personal perspective. Many women leave shared visits chatting and sharing ideas.

Shared visits are ideal for women who

- need routine follow-up care.
- want more information on health problems.
- benefit from mind-body care or more time with a physician.
- require frequent return visits.

If your health care facility offers this option, consider trying it.

Appendix 3

Managing Migraine Headaches

Hormones and Migraines

- Migraines are three times more common in women than in men.

- Hormone changes can have negative effects on migraines—and positive effects, as well.

- Most people who have headaches incorrectly diagnose themselves as having tension or sinus headaches, when they are probably common migraines.

- Treating headaches with over-the-counter medications more than three times a week may lead to more headaches.

- Keeping a headache diary can help you identify headache triggers so that you can avoid them and decrease the frequency of pain.

- Riboflavin (a B vitamin) and magnesium (a mineral) may help reduce migraines.

What Causes a Migraine?

A migraine begins when blood vessels in the brain constrict and get smaller. This happens for unknown reasons. In response to blood vessel constriction, the brain sends a message for the narrowed blood vessels to expand. Pain begins when blood vessels in the brain enlarge, causing painful throbbing in the head.

Who Gets Migraines?

Migraines usually begin in people under age 40. More women than men get migraines. Those who suffer from migraines often have close relatives who experience them. Migraine symptoms include the following:

- Throbbing pain in the head
- Localized pain on one side of the head that spreads to the whole head
- Loss of appetite, nausea, vomiting
- Sensitivity to light and/or noise

Classic Migraines

Prior to headache pain and other symptoms, about 15 to 20 percent of migraine sufferers experience an aura or warning. An aura is a vision-related sign that develops over five to twenty minutes and can include the following:

- Blind spots
- Complete loss of vision in one eye

- Seeing flashing lights and zigzag lines
- Shape and size distortion

Migraine Triggers

Stress Letdown

The body produces more adrenaline during stressful times, and this narrows blood vessels. When stress diminishes, the arteries relax and expand. Expansion of the brain's arteries can result in migraine headaches.

Ovulation or Menstruation

Hormone fluctuations during menstrual cycles can trigger migraines. Menstrual migraines may get worse in perimenopause, and such migraines usually get better after menopause. Some women on cycled hormones (whether for contraception or hormone therapy) get worse. Keeping hormone levels constant can help reduce or eliminate the hormone withdrawal headache that many women experience.

Dieting/Fasting

Skipping meals lowers blood sugar levels, which triggers migraines.

Caffeine

An unusual drop in caffeine intake may allow the brain's blood vessels to relax and trigger a migraine.

Diet

Some migraine sufferers find that certain foods trigger migraines. These include the following:

- Aged cheeses/pizza
- Luncheon meats
- Sausages or hot dogs
- Onions
- Chocolate
- Yogurt
- MSG (found in some Asian food)

Medication and Alcohol

Alcohol and some medications can cause excessive expansion of arteries with resulting migraines.

Weather Changes

Change in barometric pressure can trigger migraines.

Migraine Prevention

- Eat three meals a day and don't skip breakfast. If you sleep in on weekends, start getting up at your normal weekday time.
- Maintain routine bed and wake times.
- Develop hobbies and activities that relieve everyday stress.
- Exercise regularly to help the body be less sensitive to factors that trigger migraines.
- Keep migraine medication on hand.

Migraine Treatment

Vitamins

Magnesium can be helpful along with B-complex vitamins, specifically riboflavin and pyridoxine (B_6).

Preventive Medications

Beta blockers can keep arteries relaxed. Nonsteroidal drugs can decrease inflammation.

Abortive Medications

Taken at the onset of migraine attacks, these medications narrow expanded blood vessels and relieve pain. They may be combined with antinauseants and pain relievers to treat other migraine symptoms. There are several triptans, such as the IMITREX tablets, nasal spray, and injections, and other products, including the RELPAX tablet (which acts only on the cerebral vessels), oral FROVA (for menstrual migraines), and ZOMIG (available in oral and sublingual—under-the-tongue—tablets as well as nasal spray). TOPAMAX (topiramate) is approved to reduce migraine headaches and in some women is associated with weight loss.

Biofeedback Therapy

Biofeedback equipment helps patients learn to identify stressful situations and control their bodies' reactions to them. It is combined with psychotherapy and often decreases the need for medications.

Appendix 4

Caregiving Keys

Whether you're caring for an aging parent or spouse, the responsibilities of caring for a loved one can weaken your own health if you're not careful. Many women find themselves "sandwiched" between the needs of older relatives and younger children. Consider these tips to help you manage the job:

- **Stay informed.** Learn all you can about aging and the specific medical conditions that your loved one is dealing with. Check into available community resources by calling your area hospital or asking your physician for references. Support groups can help you manage your caregiving role and link you with other women confronting similar challenges.

- **Ask for help.** Have regular family meetings and update out-of-town people by phone and email so that they understand the situation. Don't assume that all of them know what is going on; unless you tell them, they won't know you need help. Involve the person you are caring for in the decisions that affect him or her and encourage as much independence as possible. Remember, it's okay for you to say no. And check into home services, such as Home Instead Senior Care, which can provide helpful services to your loved one.

- **Take care of yourself.** If you don't care for yourself, how will you care for your loved one? Eat balanced meals, take time to exercise, and participate in relaxing activities. Use respite services or ask a family member to support you so you can take time out. Keep in touch with friends and close relatives—don't isolate yourself during this difficult time. While it may seem overwhelming to be the caregiver and keep up with your social life, the outlet will serve as an important diversion from caregiving stress. Review your work and stress level monthly and discuss your situation with a third party if necessary—a physician or counselor.

- **Accept your emotions.** Frustration, sadness, anger, and fear are emotions that come with the job of caregiving. Accept them without guilt. Perfection is not an option—and you're doing the best you possibly can for your loved one. Seek support from caregiver programs in your community or lean on a trusted friend or family member. Don't bottle up your emotions and stress.

Plan for Caregiving

You can't completely plan for caregiving, but you can prepare resources and gather information that will help you when the time comes to make choices about your loved one's care. Always include your parents or spouse in these conversations—ask them about their concerns with aging, their preferences for an ideal situation, and their specific wishes about legal and financial issues.

Here are some conversations you'll want to have with your loved ones.

- **Who are the friends and contacts?** To whom does your loved one turn in an emergency—a friend, neighbor, family member? Make a list of these people and their phone numbers.

- **What are the housing preferences?** Has your loved one considered living somewhere besides his or her current home? Would moving into your home be an acceptable option—especially if this means leaving another city or state? What about assisted-living facilities or group home settings? What about the option of downsizing or moving into a more manageable space in a condo or apartment?

- **What is the financial situation?** Don't wait to talk about money, one of the most difficult topics to address. Be aware of income sources such as Social Security and pensions, bank accounts and investments—including those that are jointly owned with a child or other family member—and assets such as antiques or collections. Be aware of credit cards and watch for unusual activity after an illness or accident.

- **What is the medical history?** Are there medical conditions or health problems that you don't know about? Which medications does your loved one take? Contact the appropriate physicians if your loved one cannot answer these questions. Who is the health insurance provider, and are there restrictions on receiving health care or requirements for emergency care away from home?

- **What legal documents are missing?** Does your loved one have a will, an advance directive such as a living will, and a health care proxy form? What about trusts and powers of attorney? Where does your loved one keep documents such as birth certificates, armed forces discharge papers, the deed to the home, and insurance policies? You'll want to find out this information—and be sure that the will is up-to-date.

Create a Caregiver Resource

It's a good idea to put together a notebook with critical information. This guidebook can serve as a manual for other family members helping with caregiving, and it also helps keep all records in one place. Here are some suggestions on documents you'll want to keep in this notebook (adapted from the Western Reserve Area Agency on Aging, Cleveland, Ohio, *www.psa10a.org*).

- Emergency contact information
- A copy of the durable power of attorney and any medical advance directives
- Insurance information regarding Medicare, Medicaid, an HMO, or supplemental insurance
- Names, telephone numbers, and addresses of friends and clergy
- Health care contacts, including doctors and their specialties, hospital preference or limitations, and pharmacy information
- A schedule of a typical day to guide a substitute caregiver
- A short biography of your loved one which can provide a substitute caregiver with topics of conversation.

Appendix 5

A Word on Compounding Pharmacies

In the wake of the Women's Health Initiative, women have been (inappropriately) told that all traditional prescription hormones are risky, and they have therefore turned to alternatives. Women have been hoodwinked when they've been told that "natural bio-identical hormones compounded individually are safer and risk-free." Any hormone, including those hormones mixed on the premises by a compounding pharmacist, carries potential risks.

Quality, purity, safety, and efficacy are not monitored at compounding pharmacies, and that is of great concern. I see women who want to avoid any risk of HT taking unmonitored substances and putting themselves at greater risk!

All compounded hormones begin with chemically synthesized hormone powders, and when you visit these "customized compounding pharmacies," you don't know how much or exactly what you are receiving.

The way the media, the National Institutes of Health, and many physicians and patients handled the results of the WHI study made the situation ripe for charlatans, marketers, and snake oil salespeople to take advantage of menopausal women in need of symptom relief, promising them great benefits with no risk. Be wary of anything that sounds too good to be true. And do not order hormones in the form of creams or pills over the Internet.

I do prescribe some medications that have to be compounded, but by and large I favor commercially available hormone products since they have been rigorously tested and meet FDA safety standards.

Do not assume that because you get treatments from a compounding pharmacy that they've been proven effective and safe.

The FDA has approved many forms and doses of prescription hormone therapy for treatment of menopause symptoms. You need to find a trusted physician who will work with you to regulate dosages and assess treatment effects as opposed to someone who is out to make a personal profit from your misery.

Appendix 6

Resources for Midlife Women

Websites

- Cleveland Clinic Center for Specialized Women's Health:
  www.clevelandclinic.org/womenshealth/

- American Academy of Sleep Medicine SleepEducation.com:
  www.sleepeducation.com

- American Dietetic Association:
  www.eatright.org

- National Osteoporosis Foundation:
  www.nof.org

- Speaking of Women's Health:
  www.speakingofwomenshealth.com

- The North American Menopause Society:
  www.menopause.org

- U.S. Department of Agriculture MyPyramid.gov:
  www.mypyramid.gov

- U.S. Department of Healthy & Human Services
  Dietary Guidelines for Americans:
  www.health.gov/dietaryguidelines

Suggested Books

Aronne, Louis J., MD. *Weigh Less, Live Longer: Dr. Lou Aronne's "Getting Healthy" Plan for Permanent Weight Control.* New York: John Wiley & Sons, 1996.

Foldvary-Shaefer, Nancy, DO., *The Cleveland Clinic Guide to Sleep Disorders.* New York: Kaplan, 2009.

Peeke, Pamela, MD., *Body for Life for Women: A Woman's Plan for Physical and Mental Transformation.* Emmaus, PA: Rodale, 2005.

Sheehy, Gail. *Sex and the Seasoned Woman: Pursuing the Passionate Life.* New York: Ballantine, 2007.

Index

About the Cleveland Clinic
Center for Specialized Women's Health

At the Cleveland Clinic Center for Specialized Women's Health where I practice, our "one-stop shop" includes women's health specialists (medical and surgical), social workers, specialized breast imagers, and wonderful nurses. This interdisciplinary approach in a female-friendly environment offers easy access to a suite of specialty services and allows women to see a team of specialists under one roof.

The Women's Health Center, established in 2002 at the Women's Health and Breast Pavilion with a $2 million grant from the Avon Foundation, is the product of constant evolution in the medical world. The creation of a pavilion of health services dedicated solely to women is a tribute to those who have been fighting for years to have women's health needs recognized and understood as *not* identical to men's.

Not every medical institution can offer this arrangement, and not every woman needs a suite of specialists. For those who do have such a need, our Center is a comforting space where women can express their intimate concerns to physicians and nurses, and receive medical *and* emotional support. My patients feel as if we're advocates for their health—and we are!

Holly L. Thacker, MD, FACP, CCD
Director, Center for Specialized Women's Health
Women's Health Institute
Cleveland Clinic
www.clevelandclinic.org/womenshealth/
Associate Professor of Surgery, Cleveland Clinic Lerner College
    of Medicine at Case Western Reserve University
Executive Director, Speaking of Women's Health
www.speakingofwomenshealth.com

About the Author

Holly L. Thacker, MD, a trailblazer in women's health, founded the interdisciplinary Center for Specialized Women's Health at Cleveland Clinic and one of the first women's health fellowships in the United States. Her interests include menopause and hormone therapy regimens, menstrual disorders, osteoporosis, and use of hormone therapy in breast cancer survivors. She has served as a co-investigator of various hormone therapy system regimens and osteoporosis therapeutic drug trials, and she is regarded as a national thought leader in women's health. She has published and lectured extensively on the topic of menopause and is a NAMS-credentialed Menopause Clinician.

She has chaired the annual "Speaking of Women's Health" Cleveland events for several years, received numerous health awards, and appeared on local and national television to comment on women's health.